BOTOX

and

BEYOND

YOUR GUIDE TO SAFE,
NONSURGICAL, COSMETIC PROCEDURES

BOTOX

and

BEYOND

JEROME POTOZKIN, M.D.

Advantage®

Published by Advantage, Charleston, South Carolina.
Member of Advantage Media Group.

ADVANTAGE is a registered trademark, and the Advantage colophon is a trademark of Advantage Media Group, Inc.

Printed in the United States of America.

10 9 8 7 6 5 4 3 2 1

ISBN: 978-1-64225-001-5
LCCN: 2018961608

Book design by Melanie Cloth.

This publication is designed to provide accurate and authoritative information in regard to the subject matter covered. It is sold with the understanding that the publisher is not engaged in rendering legal, accounting, or other professional services. If legal advice or other expert assistance is required, the services of a competent professional person should be sought.

Advantage Media Group is proud to be a part of the Tree Neutral® program. Tree Neutral offsets the number of trees consumed in the production and printing of this book by taking proactive steps such as planting trees in direct proportion to the number of trees used to print books. To learn more about Tree Neutral, please visit **www.treeneutral.com.**

Advantage Media Group is a publisher of business, self-improvement, and professional development books and online learning. We help entrepreneurs, business leaders, and professionals share their Stories, Passion, and Knowledge to help others Learn & Grow. Do you have a manuscript or book idea that you would like us to consider for publishing? Please visit **advantagefamily.com** or call **1.866.775.1696**.

This book is dedicated to my parents Joseph and Shondell Potozkin, my sister Amy, my amazing wife Monica, and two boys—Samuel and David—who keep me striving to be a better doctor and a better person. These amazing people have been a source of love, support, and inspiration throughout my life.

Table of Contents

Introduction

⟿

When Sally came into PotozkinMD Skincare Center, my practice in Danville, California, she had a large crusting scab on her entire left upper cheek. A forty-eight-year-old, high-level sales executive for a national company, Sally had been concerned about the signs of aging she'd noticed in her face, so she'd previously gone to one of those "med spas," or "medi spas," that are popping up everywhere.

The people inside all wore white coats and looked professional. Sally went into a room with a nurse, who told her that while the nurse would be performing the filler injection that would give her a more refreshed look, a doctor was supervising the facility. What she wasn't told was that the "supervising physician" was a rectal surgeon with no aesthetic training and was never on-site.

The nurse injected filler into her upper cheek, just underneath her eyelid. Without realizing it, though, the nurse either compressed or injected into a blood vessel, which led to the cheek being deprived of its blood supply and ulcerating into the open, bleeding sore I'd see later. Despite what Sally had been assured, the "supervising physician" couldn't help her, because he was in his office one hundred miles from the med spa facility, and the nurse was out of her league in trying to handle the problem. "Sorry, we can't help you," the nurse told her. She left Sally to treat it herself, and the result was the nasty scab on her otherwise pleasant face.

Unfortunately, Sally's experience isn't unusual. The same scenario plays out all over the country. What happened to Sally is happening to others nationwide and has only increased in prevalence since she visited me eight years ago.

Nowadays, everyone wants to be a dermatologist. That's because minimally invasive cosmetic procedures are becoming big business. The American Society for Dermatologic Surgery reported there were over four million such procedures performed in their annual 2017 survey.

There are a lot more minimally invasive procedures being performed compared to big facial cosmetic surgeries. That's partly because people are busy.

That means there are a lot more minimally invasive procedures being performed compared to big, facial cosmetic surgeries. That's partly because people are busy. They don't want the downtime associated with surgery. For some people, it's not only the cost of the procedure that matters, but the cost of being off work or away from the activities they love doing for two weeks. Plus, more invasive procedures bring greater risks. When you introduce general anesthesia, that creates a whole new risk category.

Minimally invasive procedures have advanced so far that they can really make a noticeable difference and produce great results.

The combination of people's desire—particularly baby boomers and post-baby boomers who are still super active—to look their best and look the way they feel, pressure from the job market, and advances and greater availability of different minimally invasive procedures and treatments have created a perfect storm of demand for these great, get-in/get-out procedures.

But it has also created a market where a lot of people jump into performing the procedures simply because of the money—even those whose medical training doesn't line up with these procedures. They're getting into it strictly for financial gain.

According to the industry website, Medical Spa MD, there were more than 2,100 medical spas operating in the United States in 2016. Perhaps not all of them perform filler injections, but certainly many of them do. And in many—or most—of them, the person doing the injection, whether it's a nurse, a urologist, an internal medicine specialist, or another medical professional, relies on the training they got during a weekend seminar where the instructor told them to insert the needle here, and here, and here, and not much beyond that.

A urologist deals with the kidney, bladder, and prostate. That has nothing to do with facial and body cosmetics.

California laws prevent a nurse from owning a med spa and hiring a physician to act as supervisor; a med spa practice has to be physician owned. But nurses partner with physicians in shady deals where, on paper, the practice looks like it's physician owned, but the nurse is the one who actually owns the facility.

Obviously, that's what was occurring at the facility Sally visited.

I saw this trend coming years ago—in the mid-2000s—when I was training other doctors on the use of a particular cosmetic laser. These doctors would come to my office and spend a day with me. But many of them had no business using the laser in the first place. A urologist or an anesthesiologist doesn't have the background to do these treatments.

One anesthesiologist who came in had purchased a laser but had no clue about dermatology and what the devices do. Such a practitioner can laser over skin cancers and not even know it, making them much more difficult to diagnose later. If there's a melanoma and you laser over it and remove some of the pigment, it makes it almost impossible to diagnose until the cancer grows, potentially to the point where it has already metastasized and spread to other parts of the body. If the person doing the laser treatments hadn't lasered over the spot, the melanoma could have been diagnosed right off the bat.

So it's not only a high rate of complications that these med spas present, it's also the potential for doing real harm.

I didn't want to be complicit in that. I told the laser company, "From now on, I am only training dermatologists and plastic surgeons."

As they did with Sally, these "professionals" mislead people about their credentials and education and offer services at a discount, which makes them appealing to people looking for savings on nonsurgical, cosmetic enhancement. People are trying to save a few bucks—and at best, that's about all they'll save—so they go into those lower-cost med spas where the person doing the injection is undertrained.

But I've found that most of the time, you get what you pay for. That seems to be a universal principle no matter what you're buying.

These cosmetic procedures are not commodities; they're dependent on the skill of the person delivering the procedure. Too frequently, the financial savings are not worth it—and aren't even actual savings in the long run, as Sally and many others have discovered.

Performing these noninvasive procedures looks deceptively easy; compared to a complex kidney operation, for example, it might not look that hard. So these people believe they can do it because it's just sticking in a needle and pressing the plunger, right?

No.

There's a lot more to it than what you might see on the surface. Injecting fillers and Botox and using energy-based devices for rejuvenation is highly dependent on technique. If you don't know the underlying anatomy and you're just injecting stuff into people's faces, you don't know the structures you really need to be super careful to avoid. And you can't get that knowledge by taking a weekend course.

Undertrained practitioners can overdo the injections or botch the procedure, leaving people with distorted features—or more extreme damage.

I've seen people walking around with weird-looking brows, or strange expressions on their faces. You've probably seen it, too: the "over-Botoxed" look that gives Botox a bad name.

Undertrained practitioners can overdo the injections or botch the procedure, leaving people with distorted features—or more extreme damage.

When Botox is overdone, it can look really bizarre. There are all kinds of things that can go wrong with Botox. But when it's done correctly, you can get amazing results that give a refreshed, more relaxed appearance.

For most people, as they age, their lips thin. If you can give them a little replenishment of their lost volume, it can make a big difference. Filler injections like Sally got are even more dependent on technique than Botox. If filler is injected too superficially, you can see blue lumps under the skin. The patient's face can look distorted. The most common complication that people will notice comes from overdone, overly fat lips.

And there are other risks, which I'll address in this book.

One of Sally's friends was a patient of mine. She recommended me to Sally, which is why a week later, Sally came to my office seeking help in dealing with the ulceration. Never mind about looking younger. She didn't even care about that anymore.

Sally was embarrassed when we sat down to talk about her problem, because she felt she should have known better than to go to a low-cost storefront med spa. But she really hadn't understood the nurse's lack of credentials until after the damage was done.

I assured her there was no reason to be embarrassed and that we could fix the damage—with time.

I knew exactly what the problem was when I saw the location and degree of damage to the skin. It was sitting right over an area where there's a little artery that comes out of the skull. That vessel had either been compressed or injected directly into.

Either way, it was bad.

I don't know anything about the nurse who did the injection except that she was clearly undertrained.

By the time Sally came to me in 2010, I'd already been doing injections for more than fifteen years. More importantly, I'd been thoroughly trained; after graduating from the University of Pennsylvania in 1984, I went to New York University School of Medicine, where the first thing they taught me was anatomy. I learned all the anatomical structures in the head, neck, and body, where nerves come in, where arteries come in, areas that a practitioner really needed to be careful of or avoid entirely with a needle.

That got emphasized again during my residency in dermatology at the renowned NYU Skin & Cancer Unit. Any residency in dermatology, plastic surgery, facial plastic surgery, or oculoplastic surgery emphasizes the anatomy to avoid just the sort of thing that had happened to Sally.

After my residency, I did a fellowship at the University of California, San Francisco, in a procedure called Mohs Micrographic Surgery, a precise surgical technique used to treat skin cancer. Again, I studied the anatomy, reviewing it and applying it to the different procedures I performed.

Education for the injector (the person doing the injection) is important for a number of reasons. It's important to know the different skin types to be able to treat people safely and effectively, whether you're using a laser or light-based technology. It's also important to know how to treat complications.

But at those weekend courses, you don't have time to study anatomy. And if the person doing the injection hasn't previously studied anatomy of the face, they simply won't have that knowledge of what veins and structures to avoid.

As they say, "You need to learn how to crawl before you can run." In this case, studying the anatomy of the face was crawling—and these people were trying to run first.

The truth is, there can always be complications. People get struck by lightning, and complications happen in the best of hands. I've had complications of my own—sometimes things happen—but not with the same frequency and not because of neglect.

It's not that complications don't happen with people who are highly trained; it's that they're statistically less likely to happen. And if they do happen, we know how to treat the problem.

In Sally's case, I knew how to treat the complications she'd experienced elsewhere. I told her that her healing was going to be a gradual process. Because the wound looked infected, I put some antibacterial ointment on it and told her she'd have to keep applying it herself.

It's not that complications don't happen with people who are highly trained; it's that they're statistically less likely to happen.

For a month, she had to go to all her professional and sales meetings feeling self-conscious about the dressing over her cheek.

But that wasn't the end of her treatment. The wound left a scar, which I then treated with a couple of different lasers until the scarring became almost invisible. In all, the treatment took nine months.

Going to that low-cost med spa cost her far more money and time in the end than if she'd just come to my office in the first place—or the office of any other board-certified dermatologist, plastic surgeon, oculoplastic surgeon, or facial plastic surgeon. And now she looked the same as before she'd entered that spa.

That's a painful lesson Sally learned and, hopefully, one this book can help you avoid. The good news is that there are highly trained specialists who know what they're doing and can minimize your risk from an injection or laser treatment. There are even highly trained and excellent nurse injectors working with proper supervision.

As for Sally, we finally healed her face, but by then she was reluctant to try the procedure again. After another three months, she worked up the courage, and I injected her with a filler called Restylane. All fillers have slightly different characteristics, and for that area, Restylane was the one I typically get the best results with, based on my years of experience. (See Chapter 2 for more about Restylane and other fillers.)

This time, the results were great—no problems. She looked fresher, more relaxed, less tired.

The lesson: When considering a nonsurgical cosmetic enhancement, people should worry less about the cost of the procedure and more about the person they choose to do the procedure. While practitioners use similar devices for the same procedures, the results aren't always similar, and the difference lies in who does the procedure. Selecting a provider with the proper training and experience (and an aesthetic eye) is the most important part of deciding to get a procedure.

The upside of the popularity of nonsurgical enhancements is that there are so many innovations happening in this space. People have so many different options and are much better off now than they were ten—or even five—years ago. When I was doing my residency, there were two lasers available. Now there are multiple laser companies and non-laser companies with multiple devices on the market. When I finished training, there was no Botox. It was just injectable collagen; now there are many different injections available. You'll learn about those in Chapter 1.

There are now so many people who are highly skilled and highly trained throughout the country, so why not go to one of them? After all, your face is the first thing people notice about you. If you're going to invest in making it look more refreshed or young, you deserve to get the best value for your investment. You will definitely get that from appropriately trained injectors.

That's what this book is about: educating you about your non-invasive cosmetic options and how to minimize your risk from such procedures. Hopefully, it will help you get your procedure in the safest, most effective way with the best results.

Chapter 1

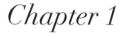

THE MAGIC OF BOTOX AND FRIENDS

Jill was in her mid-forties and feeling increased competition in the job market. Making it worse, she worked in a field where it seemed her competitors were getting younger every year.

So she came to PotozkinMD Skincare Center to spruce up her look.

"What can I do to look better?" she asked. She didn't have a specific request in mind, but with just one look it was obvious to me what the issue was. She had deep lines between her brows (we call that "the 11s," or glabella frown lines), and those lines gave her a permanent scowl. (The 11s, by the way, is probably the most common area where people get Botox.)

Those type of lines are called dynamic lines and are caused by natural facial movement. When the muscles underneath the skin contract during facial expressions, it causes the skin to pull and fold. We all do it, but the long-term effect is more pronounced for some people than others, with the result that they look like they're frowning all the time, like Jill.

If not for the scowl, which made her look mad all the time, she would have looked friendly. But the scowl probably wasn't helping her win over new clients, adding another advantage for her competitors.

For people with shallow lines, Botox works well to solve that problem by relaxing the muscles underneath the skin, thus eliminating the creasing that causes those lines. But in Jill's case, the lines were deep, and we needed to lift the lines in addition to smoothing out the muscle, so I recommended a combination of Botox and filler.

Another benefit of combining Botox with filler: immediate results. It usually takes a week for the impacts of the Botox injection to kick in, at which time patients notice that when they try to contract those muscles, not much happens. But the filler lifts the lines up right away, producing a noticeable result with a softened crease.

After the Botox took effect, along with the effects of the filler, Jill looked more relaxed. The scowling lines between her eyes were gone, and she looked like a friendly person you'd want to do business with. She told me people were responding to her differently and her sales numbers had gone up since the procedure.

She continued coming back every four months for repeat Botox injections, but she only needed repeat filler injections once every year. (There's more about fillers in Chapter 2.)

While that was a story about Botox, the same could have been said of any of the FDA-approved neuromodulators such as Botox, Dysport, or Xeomin. "Neuromodulators" is probably a new term for you, but it's not a new concept. Botox is like the Kleenex of neuromodulation—it's a brand name that is often used in place of the general category, like when people ask for a Kleenex when they really just want any tissue.

Botox is the Kleenex, and neuromodulators are the tissue. Dysport is the Puffs, and Xeomin is the Scotties.

But what are neuromodulators? They're a group of botulinum toxin type A injectable proteins that relax muscles. To get even more specific: neurons insert into a muscle and tell it to contract by secreting acetylcholine across the synapse (the space in between the nerve and the muscle). When the

Botox is like the Kleenex of neuromodulation—it's a brand name that is often used in place of the general category, like when people ask for a Kleenex when they really just want any tissue.

muscle contracts, the skin folds over. If you do it enough, the skin becomes like a piece of paper that you've folded over and over and over again.

Neuromodulators block the release of that acetylcholine, and that prevents the muscle from contracting and causing the skin to fold.

Think of it like a mute button on a telephone. If I were speaking to you on the phone and telling you to do something, but first I hit the mute button, nothing would get done, because you wouldn't hear a word of what I was saying. That's how neuromodulators work—they prevent the muscles from hearing that they're supposed to contract.

If you stop folding that piece of paper, put it under a book, and you come back a minute later, then the crease is still there. But if you come back after two weeks, the crease is much softer.

That's how neuromodulators work.

Interestingly, one of the newer findings with Botox is that it can help people who suffer from depression. We are not exactly sure how, but many, many studies have shown this to be the case.[1] It might be because these patients have a more relaxed appearance, so people they come into contact with respond to them differently. That might also explain why some of my patients who are in sales have reported to me that their sales numbers have gone up since receiving Botox treatments.

Botox for cosmetic purposes was an accidental discovery; like a lot of things in medicine, it's not being used now for what it was originally intended for. Originally it was used for treating a condition called blepharospasm—where someone has twitchy eyelids.

---

1   TH Kruger and MA Wollmer, "Depression--An emerging indication for botulinum toxin treatment," *Toxicon* 107, Pt A (December 2015): 154–7, https://doi.org/10.1016/j.toxicon.2015.09.035; K Maasumi et al., "Effect of Onabotulinumtoxin A Injection on Depression in Chronic Migraine," *Headache* 55, no. 9 (October 2015): 1218–24, https://doi.org/10.1111/head.12657; A Zamanian et al., "Efficacy of Botox versus Placebo for Treatment of Patients with Major Depression," *Iran J Public Health* 46, no. 7 (July 2017): 982–4; BE Demiryurek et al., "Effects of onabotulinumtoxinA treatment on efficacy, depression, anxiety, and disability in Turkish patients with chronic migraine," *Neurol Sci* 37, no. 11 (November 2016): 1779–84, https://doi.org/10.1007/s10072-016-2665-z; AK Parsaik et al., "Role of Botulinum Toxin in Depression," *J Psychiatr Pract* 22, no. 2 (March 2016): 99–110, https://doi.org/10.1097/PRA.0000000000000136.

Jean Carruthers, MD, an oculoplastic surgeon in Canada, used Botox to treat eye twitching. Her patients were coming back to her and telling her that they liked the fact that they weren't twitching anymore—but they really liked that their wrinkles were softening.

So Jean and her husband, Alistair Carruthers, MD—a dermatologist—decided to start treating different wrinkles that were caused by the pulling muscles underneath the skin.

According to the book *22 Immutable Laws of Marketing*, by Al Ries and Jack Trout, it's always better to be first to market than best in market. Botox was the first neuromodulator to market, and no one had seen anything like it. So it gained a lot of popularity—and the brand name recognition that still holds today.

In the late 1990s, I went to a conference and heard the Carruthers speak; what they said intrigued me, so I went back to my office and ordered one vial of Botox. I injected it into my nurse—who also had 11s—and within a week it was like magic. It was astonishing. The dynamic lines were softened and she was no longer frowning. She looked great, and it had the added bonus that I couldn't tell if she was angry with me.

Up until that point, the only thing we had to treat wrinkles was injectable collagen, which really did not work that well. So these Botox results were convincing.

I ordered more vials and have done thousands of injections since.

The 11s are not the only areas we inject Botox into. We also use it to treat crow's feet and lines in the upper forehead and neck, and the marionette lines around the mouth. It's also used for treating excess sweating (no kidding).

After we started offering the Botox treatments, we saw an influx of patients. We didn't even advertise. We simply started telling our patients about it, and they told other people that we offered it, and the news spread by word of mouth. People noticed it and then started coming in.

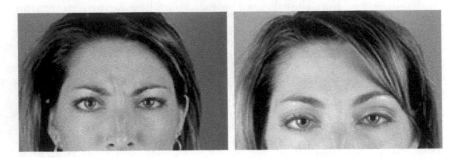

These photographs demonstrate a young woman frowning prior to Botox treatment to her glabella and then two weeks after treatment attempting to frown. After treatment there is no pull of the muscles under the skin.

For years, Botox owned the market, but in 2009, Dysport received FDA approval, and in 2010, Xeomin joined the market. All three work the same way and are botulinum toxin type A, but each one has a slightly different molecule. I won't get too technical on that, because I don't think that knowledge will really help you.

Botox is still the primary neuromodulator I use today, and it's my default, but I'll use any of the three as needed. Botox is the most expensive of the three, so sometimes a patient will prefer a less expensive treatment. Or maybe they've found that one works better for them.

Dermatologists performed over 2.1 million neuromodulator treatments in 2017, according to the American Society of Dermatologic Surgery's annual 2017 survey, while the American Society of Aesthetic Plastic Surgery reported their members performing about 1.6 million neuromodulator procedures in 2017.

Among those getting Botox treatment is my older sister, Amy. An all-natural, Berkeley kind of woman, she resisted getting injections because she believed in natural looks. But as time progressed, I noticed her lines getting deeper and deeper. So did some of her friends, who started telling her, "Hey, you should really go see your brother and have him treat that for you." She came in for an injection one time, and she was so happy with the natural-looking results that for the last ten years she has come in every four to six months like clockwork.

The truth is, the results aren't always so good. Sometimes, as I mentioned in the introduction, it's done by people who don't know exactly what they're doing. With neuromodulators, the technique is important; you need to know the underlying anatomy, because you're not injecting the wrinkle, you're injecting the muscle under the skin that's causing the wrinkle. The goal with Botox is to create a natural, relaxed appearance. The goal is not to paralyze someone's face and have them look frozen.

We've all seen that—when someone's face looks motionless. That's a result of too much Botox. Or maybe they have brows that go up and look strange like Jack Nicholson's. Or maybe their face droops. That's overdoing the Botox, as well.

Because the effects of the Botox take a week to kick in, the patient leaves the treatment unaware that they got a bad injection or that they may require a slight adjustment a week or so later. It's only later that they discover the mistake. Sometimes it isn't a mistake but simply that some people are more sensitive to the effects.

We've all seen that—when someone's face looks motionless. That's a result of too much Botox.

Unfortunately, we're seeing a trend of unqualified people performing this procedure … poorly. And that's often (but not always) because the person doing the injections doesn't know enough about the underlying anatomy of the face.

I see people who have obviously had Botox, and I am sure you have, too. Their face looks a little weird. I wonder: Why would they do that when there are many highly trained, skilled people available to inject them properly so that it looks good? Is it to save $25 to $50? Honestly, it doesn't make sense to me to do that; they're better off not doing anything than saving a handful of bucks and looking strange.

The good thing and the bad thing about Botox is that it's not permanent. If you get Botox and it looks weird, in about four months the effects will disappear.

So, how can the person doing the injection make sure they're not over-injecting? Because it takes seven days to kick in, there is no way to see at the time of injection if you've put in enough. The injector has to know how to dose it and where to inject it, because there's no immediate feedback.

My experience has given me a feel for how much Botox to put into a person's face. Of course, everyone is different, so if I'm injecting for the first time, I err on the side of caution. I'll put in less than what I think is the maximum amount they should get and encourage the patient to come back in two to four weeks to make sure it's doing what we want it to do. If they need an adjustment, I'm always happy to put in more without charge.

Because once you put it in, you can't take it out. You just have to wait.

Unfortunately, undertrained injectors aren't the only worry. Unethical providers pose a risk to patients, too.

Sometimes, to save money, a clinic will use Botox imported from another country, which is illegal. Or they will use fake Botox.

In November 2004, Dr. Eric Kaplan and his wife, Bonnie, of Palm Beach Gardens, Florida, went to a local clinic for Botox injections. They were treated by an osteopath whose license had been suspended. This individual injected them with research-grade botulinum toxin obtained from a California company that makes anthrax, cholera, and diphtheria for medical research.

The couple may have received almost three thousand times the estimated lethal dose of the toxin, according to a report in the *Journal of the American Medical Association*.[2] They got botulism—which can cause paralysis and death—but they survived.

More recently, in 2017, a nurse was fired from a med spa for refusing to give fake injections.[3]

If you find a place with cheap Botox (or Dysport or Xeomin) treatments: beware. They may be using imported or fake Botox, and then you have no idea what you're actually getting injected into your face.

We want to trust our medical providers. We want to believe they have our best interests at heart. But whenever money's to be made or money's to be saved, you have to be really careful.

How can you be careful? You want to make sure you go to a legitimate, board-certified physician, preferably in dermatology, plastic surgery, oculoplastic surgery, or ENT (ear, nose, and throat). No two faces are exactly the same, and someone who's board-certified in one of those areas is more likely to have an understanding of the underlying facial anatomy, how muscles work, and what to inject where. They're more likely to get you a safe and great result. If

---

2   "Botox Treatment: Make Sure It's the Real Thing," New York Times, November 23, 2006. https://www.nytimes.com/2006/11/23/fashion/23botulism.html.

3   Liz Ritter, "Nurse Fired After Refusing to Inject Fake Botox," New Beauty, October 11, 2016, https://www.newbeauty.com/hottopic/blogpost/9959-fake-botox-meant-for-animals.

something needs an adjustment, they're more likely to know exactly how to make that adjustment—just how much Botox to put in and where.

If you go to a reputable board-certified specialist (I happen to know a pretty good one), you won't be injected with some off-label fake or counterfeit Botox. And you can be sure they know what they're doing.

Make sure you see their certification in dermatology, plastic surgery, facial plastic surgery, or oculoplastic surgery before getting any procedure done.

The difference is in training, as I discussed in the Introduction. On top of that, I personally guarantee every neuromodulation treatment that I do. If a patient needs an adjustment on their treatment within a month of injections, I do that adjustment for free.

CHAPTER TAKEAWAYS:

- The two biggest fears I see from patients when we talk about Botox:

    1. That they will look strange

    2. That it's not safe for them

- When Botox is done properly, the results can be phenomenal.

- Botox can soften wrinkles and create a more relaxed expression—it can look natural and not frozen.

- If the person doing your injections is undertrained, the results might look strange and the procedure may be unsafe. Any medical procedure has potential side effects, but neuromodulation is a safe procedure if done by a professional.

Chapter 2

~

FILLERS, OR THE SINGLE REASON YOU MIGHT NOT NEED A FACE-LIFT

People—primarily women—come to my office because they know they need something done to fight off the effects of time. They don't like what they see in the mirror, and they look tired and older than they feel. They want to look better. They don't want to look different from who they are, but they want to look like the best natural version of themselves. They're often not sure what they need, but they know they want something to help them look more rested and more youthful.

But when I suggest a dermal filler injection as a way to refresh their look, they'll say, "Oh, I was injected with Juvederm and it didn't work" or "I was injected with Restylane and it didn't work."

Or they'll mention a friend of theirs who had an exaggerated, over-puffy look after a filler injection. They may think about someone they've seen out and about in town who had been overtreated and whose facial features had ended up distorted. Maybe the problem was the lips or the cheek, but something just didn't look right. They're used to seeing celebrities like Meg Ryan or Lisa Rinna, whose lips have been really distorted, and those are the images in their head.

And they're partially right—if it's obvious that you've done something, you're better off not doing anything.

But just to be clear: in most cases, it's not that the filler didn't work; it's that the injection wasn't done properly.

According to the American Society of Dermatologic Surgery, their members performed 1.64 million soft tissue filler procedures in 2017. The American Society for Aesthetic Plastic Surgery report about 723,000 for the same time period—but you don't see two million people walking around with overripe lips or bloated cheeks.

SOFT-TISSUE FILLERS
Procedure Totals 2012-2017

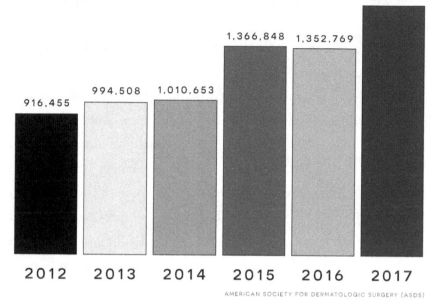

AMERICAN SOCIETY FOR DERMATOLOGIC SURGERY (ASDS)

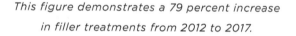

*This figure demonstrates a 79 percent increase
in filler treatments from 2012 to 2017.*

Most people don't talk to others about getting filler injections. I've had patients mention a friend of theirs who is also a patient of ours, who we know is getting filler treatments in our office, and my patient says something like "You know, I can't believe so-and-so. She looks so great and she's not doing anything. She's just all natural." Everything that happens in our office is strictly confidential, so I don't say anything. But that friend—and the majority of the two million who got a filler treatment last year—is an example of how natural filler injections can look when done well.

But that's often the big barrier I have to overcome when recommending filler injections. My method for overcoming it is simple: I gesture to one of my assistants who is standing in the room, and I ask, "Does Stephanie look weird or strange to you?"

"No, she looks great."

"Well, this recommended procedure is what Stephanie has done."

(Most of my staff receive injections. It's a perk of the job, as well as walking examples of my work.)

That works well to overcome patients' hesitancy. I've managed to replace the image of overdone or poorly done injections with a successfully done one, and it changes the patient's opinion of the treatment.

> *I've managed to replace the image of overdone or poorly done injections with a successfully done one, and it changes the patient's opinion of the treatment.*

Fillers work by ... well, filling in the face. As we age, we lose volume in our face. There's loss of bony volume around the mouth and a loss of fat volume. Fat on the face will often shrink and sink. When I inject the filler onto the bone, it fills in that volume and lifts the skin, giving the look that you've turned back the clock.

Fillers have changed dramatically since I started practicing in 1992. Back then, the only filler we had was bovine collagen—the US Food and Drug Administration approved Zyderm collagen and Zyplast collagen in 1981.

We were working then primarily to address what are called the nasolabial folds, which you can think of as the parentheses around the mouth. Even young people have those folds, so the collagen wasn't really about making people look younger. It did soften their look, though.

But there were disadvantages to collagen. It didn't really last very long, and some people had allergic reactions to it. With nonhuman collagen, there's a risk of developing an allergy and granulomas, which are inflamed areas of tissue. About four to six percent of patients develop granulomas at the injection site.

In 2004, Restylane got FDA approval. Restylane is made from hyaluronic acid, a substance that is naturally found in the body—in the eyes and joints—and had been used in Europe for several years before it was approved for use in the United States.

Then in 2006, Juvederm got approval, followed by many more hyaluronic acid fillers, which have become the most popular fillers used in the United States.

These fillers last longer than collagen and look natural when they're injected properly. There are different fillers within each brand of hyaluronic acid fillers, each with a different filling and lifting property. They differ based on their consistency and how thick they are. That creates more flexibility and options for me as the person doing the injections.

For instance, when I'm injecting a filler deep into the skin, almost on the bone, I want a robust, thicker filler that has more lifting properties. When I'm injecting into fine lines, like the vertical lip lines (which we call "smoker's lines"), I want to use a thinner filler that's designed to get into those really fine lines. If I tried to inject a bulky filler into those fine lines, they'd look lumpy and bumpy.

In 2014, filler treatments changed when we started looking at the mid-face area—the upper cheeks and areas underneath the eyes. As we age, the fat pads in that area shrink and droop, creating a hollow look underneath the eye and making the nasolabial folds deeper.

With new fillers like Voluma or Restylane Lyft, we can actually fill and lift those areas and make a big difference in making people look more youthful and well rested.

Now we can do full-face rejuvenation and fill in the hollows and the temples as people age. We're really looking at full-face correction, as opposed to just individual lines. We're able to do a lot of things we never thought could be done with fillers—things we used to think could only be done with surgery. (More on that in a little while.)

As innovations in dermal fillers advance, the results are lasting longer than ever. Some fillers in the Restylane and Juvederm family last up to a year. A single injection of Voluma lasts up to two years.

Sculptra, which is poly-L-lactic acid, also called PLLA, was originally FDA approved in 2004 for treating patients with HIV who lost fat in their face. Since then, it's gotten FDA approval for aesthetic purposes.

PLLA is a material that's found in some absorbable sutures—those self-dissolving stitches that most of us have had used on us to close a deep cut or surgical wound—and is a very different filler than the hyaluronic acid fillers. The way PLLA works is like the "pearl in the oyster" phenomena. It is injected deep in a suspension mixed with saline or sterile water and a local anesthetic, and it stimulates the body's own collagen production. If someone has a really slim, skinny face, Sculptra can reflate it like a balloon. It's kind of like going from a raisin to a grape.

Typically, we'll do three treatment sessions of Sculptra, waiting about a month in between, and see the full results at three to six months because it's the body creating its own collagen. Those results will typically last a long time, up to two years.

Another filler, Radiesse, also got approval in 2006. A more robust filler made out of calcium hydroxyapatite, it's designed to be injected deep in the cheekbones and temporal hollows, and it can actually be injected in the back of the hands—it's FDA approved for that. It's certainly not for fine lines like lips.

But early on, inexperienced practitioners injected Radiesse into the lips, leaving those patients with white nodules in their lips. Let that be a word of caution (yes, that's a recurrent theme here): There are many expert injectors throughout the country who are highly trained and know what they're doing. Be sure to see one of them for your treatment.

There are even long-lasting, or more permanent-type fillers, but that's not necessarily a good thing. In fact, time and time again, people ask me about permanent fillers, but I prefer not to inject those. I only inject into my patients what I would inject into a family member, and I would not inject these into a family member because those permanent fillers usually have tiny, polymethyl methacrylate plastic beads in them, and people can develop a long-lasting allergic reaction to those beads after injection. But then they're stuck with them unless they get that material cut out of their face.

Also, as time goes on, our face changes and there are shifts in volume. If I inject something into someone's face when they're thirty, by the time they're fifty they may have some change of volume or some sagging of the skin. That early permanent filler may have moved down, and now it sits there as a lump that's not going away.

Contrast that to the hyaluronic acid fillers, for instance. If there is a bump or nodule, or a result someone's unhappy with, we can literally melt those away by injecting an enzyme called hyaluronidase.

While I don't inject the permanent fillers, I do inject long-lasting ones like Sculptra, Voluma, and Radiesse.

With so many options available, an expert's knowledge is more important than ever. With competing filler manufacturers constantly rolling out new products, the marketplace is crowded. So the injector really needs to know the properties and best uses for each filler and be able to judge the best filler for an individual patient and for a specific area of the face. And that's the type of knowledge you can't get from a weekend training course—which presents another risk that you as a patient have to deal with.

Compared to Botox, fillers are even more technique dependent, and the risks of complications are far greater. Because of where they are injected, the potential for side effects are greater with fillers than with Botox.

With fillers, it's like Goldilocks and the three bears; you don't want too little, and you don't want too much. The goal is to put in just the right amount.

If I have to choose between too much and not enough, I would go with not enough, because I can always put in more later.

> *With fillers, it's like Goldilocks and the three bears; you don't want too little, and you don't want too much.*

Some people want that over-plump look—it's a small trend—and there are always doctors who will accommodate them. Michael Jackson had people who kept distorting him more and more. It's amazing to me that doctors kept doing stuff to him. But he had a lot of money, and money rules the world.

Those people who want that exaggerated or distorted look are not my people. To me, when women get gigantic breast implants, it doesn't look natural or aesthetically pleasing. I don't understand why people would want to do that. It's the same with filler; I don't understand why someone would want to go overboard and look distorted.

I educate people about how the right amount of filler can make them look normal—and how that's actually the point of the fillers. But if somebody still wants to overdo it despite the information I have shared with them, then I am not the best person to help them.

Earlier, I mentioned that we can now do things with fillers that we could only do with surgery before. In fact, I'll occasionally have patients who, after consultation, insist they don't want to do fillers, and that they'll just get a face-lift instead. They think a face-lift will fix their problem and then they won't have to get injections anymore. But that's not how it works, because face-lifts and fillers address two different things.

It's kind of like saying, "I'm going to redo my kitchen so that I never have to paint the exterior of my house anymore." They're not the same thing.

For example, Katie was a woman in her fifties who didn't like what she saw in the mirror, and because she had no knowledge about what fillers could do, she came in to find out the options available to her. Really, though, she wanted a referral to a plastic surgeon for a face-lift. (I don't do face-lifts.)

When I evaluated her, I noticed her lower face looked great, she had no neck fat, and her main problem was that she had lost volume. Her lips were thinner, her upper-mid face was thinner, and her temples were hollow.

I pointed out what was making her look older, and how the upper-mid cheek under her eye area had sunken in, making her eye bags look more prominent. I told her that these are not things a face-lift would help. A face-lift can do great things for someone who has a lot of sagging skin and redundancy of the neck (excess skin), but for someone who has volume loss, a face-lift will not address their concerns.

Rather than a costly face-lift that required a period of recovery, I injected her with Voluma in the upper cheek and Restylane in her lips and the tear trough, which is the area underneath the eye bag.

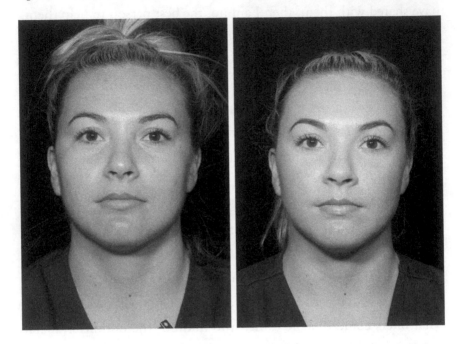

Photos show improvement of the under eye or "tear trough" area treated with injectable filler.

That course of treatment gave her everything that she wanted, and it didn't require time off work, the risk of general anesthesia, and the risk of surgery. It was a great solution for her.

Katie really just needed education. As a physician, I see myself in the role of educating people and then letting them make the decision themselves about what's best for them.

All of this is why selecting the best provider is important. I think of using injectable fillers as being a human sculptor. I'm sculpting the human face. If you were to commission a sculpture, would you commission someone who just took a weekend art course, or would you commission a master sculptor? Where do you think you'll get the better piece of art? And if the piece of art is your face, you might want to think about investing in the very best.

The most important variable in filler treatment isn't the filler that's being injected, it's the person doing the filling—the person holding the syringe—because filler treatment is highly dependent on technique and skill.

There are so many things that person—the injector—needs to know. It's not about just sticking a needle into someone's face. You have to have the scientific knowledge of the anatomy of the face, a very complicated place. There are blood vessels, there are nerves, there's bone, there's fat, and there's skin. The person doing the injection has to know the basic anatomy and the areas where they have to be cautious. They need to know what's best for the individual characteristics of a person's face, and how to evaluate that and determine the best plan of action.

The most important variable in filler treatment isn't the filler that's being injected, it's the person doing the filling—the person holding the syringe—because filler treatment is highly dependent on technique and skill.

You also want the injector to have an aesthetic eye, so they know what looks good and what will not look good proportionally.

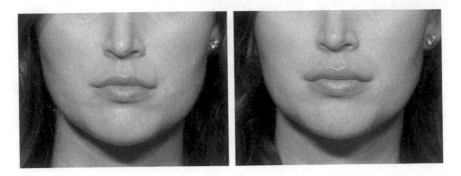

Lip filler showing subtle, natural enhancement.

Early in my career, I took sculpting classes every week at an art school in San Francisco, which really helped me visualize what I was doing as a dermatologist. I look at fillers the same way I approached those sculptures. After all, I'm just sculpting the human face on a live person. (Those clay sculptures I worked on in those classes, by the way, are still on display in my house.)

A skilled dermatologist is more likely to know the anatomy, more likely to have a better aesthetic eye, and more likely to have the judgment and skill to get you the best result possible.

With fillers, if the person doing the injection doesn't know what they're doing, or they don't know the anatomy, there's a greater risk of injecting into or near a blood vessel, causing an ulceration like Sally (from the Introduction) suffered. That ulceration, if not treated, can cause permanent scarring.

That can be a big problem.

Another reason it's important to use a skilled and highly trained injector: some facilities will import fillers from different countries, which saves them money. In the United States, you have to purchase fillers through certain FDA-approved distribution channels. Importing fillers is illegal in the United States as there is no quality control and counterfeit products are very common. Other countries, though, don't have those laws, so you never know quite what you're getting with imported filler because there is a lot of counterfeiting going on.

Those facilities then pass on the lower cost to their clients, making their services more attractive to you as the patient.

But the reason they have the lower fees is that they're importing product, and you don't know if you're getting what you're supposed to get. Even if the syringe has the product name on it, you might not be getting that product—it might be some cheap substitute because it's not coming from an FDA-approved distribution channel.

If something seems too good to be true, it probably is. If the filler injections are a great deal—cheaper than you'd anticipated—be skeptical about what is being injected into your face. Because I know the cost of the legitimate fillers, and they aren't that cheap.

If you're going to invest in refreshing your face, you want to make sure you get it done right; otherwise you're just throwing away money—or worse. You could be risking health complications.

CHAPTER TAKEAWAYS:

- In the last decade, fillers have really changed aesthetic medicine and have allowed us to turn back the clock with minimal to no downtime, avoiding general anesthesia and the risks of surgery.

- The number of filler treatments are on the rise.

- Great results are certainly obtainable.

- You want to think more about who is injecting you as opposed to what is being injected.

- Choose an expert with appropriate training, and let that

expert educate you about what's best for you. (Then you won't have to waste time online trying to find out what the best filler is for you.)

Chapter 3

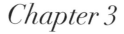

ENERGY-POWERED
REJUVENATION

K athleen was aging naturally, but she was concerned that her face had multiple, noticeably broken capillaries, brown splotches, and discolorations. She came to my office for help in erasing those marks.

Injections would be useless for that issue. Nothing needed to be pumped back up or filled out.

I recommended a treatment called intense pulsed light (IPL). IPL is a noninvasive, non-ablative resurfacing technique, meaning it targets the abnormalities of the skin without vaporizing tissue or causing a break in the skin. It works on the same principles as lasers—light energy is absorbed into specific targets in the skin. In this case, it was unwanted pigmentation and small superficial blood vessels. The light energy is converted to heat energy, which damages those targeted structures.

Unlike lasers, though, IPL systems deliver many wavelengths in each pulse of light rather than just one pure wavelength. Most IPL systems use filters to refine the energy output for the treatment of areas on the face, neck, or chest; the filters enhance penetration without using excessive energy levels and allow for targeting of specific chromophores (skin components that absorb light).

IPL technology was initially called "photoderm." It was rushed to the marketplace—something that happens too often—in the late 1990s to treat leg veins. But it didn't work for that, and patients were getting blistered and scarred, so it became unofficially known as "photoburn" among my peers. It took a while for the industry to figure out how to use this technology correctly and safely, but eventually, someone realized we could safely use it for treating vessels and brown spots on the face.

The advantage of IPL therapy is its minimal downtime; a patient can often have the procedure done and return to work the next day.

The advantage of IPL therapy is its minimal downtime; a patient can often have the procedure done and return to work the next day.

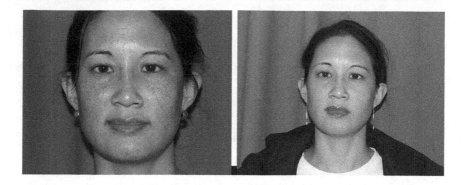

Before and after treatment with intense pulsed light for
skin rejuvenation and removal of brown spots.

Because non-ablative resurfacing isn't as intensive as ablative resurfacing—where both the dermis and epidermis are injured to produce a much more noticeable outcome—we typically do five treatments of IPL, with three weeks between each treatment.

After Kathleen's fifth treatment, she came back to the office, and she had this look on her face. It was clear she wasn't happy.

"What's the matter?" I asked.

"I don't see any difference from before I started the treatments to now," she responded.

"Hold on one second," I said. I presented her with the pictures we'd taken of her before we started treatment three months previous. I put those pictures in front of her and gave her a mirror … and her jaw dropped, because the difference was amazing. The discolorations and broken capillaries were nearly invisible now.

To me, who only saw her periodically, the difference had been apparent. But the changes that IPL brings about are gradual. So to her, who was looking in the mirror as these gradual changes intensified every day, it had seemed there had been no change at all.

And honestly, that's what we want. Since the whole purpose of what I do is to help my patients look more natural, that gradual improvement means that you don't look like you got work done during your lunch break. It's just like the trend in hair dyes, where users brush in the dye over time to create the gradual darkening of their hair so that the changes are imperceptible until they're set.

But sometimes people forget what they looked like before.

IPL is one tool in a category of energy-based devices for photo rejuvenation, which means they plug into the wall and are used to treat the skin to remove discoloration, treat wrinkles and acne scarring, erase tattoos, and tighten the skin and fine lines. Besides IPL, that category includes lasers—such as pulsed dye lasers and Fraxel lasers—radio frequency devices (which we don't use in my office, except for the device for vaginal rejuvenation that we'll talk about in Chapter 5), and micro-pulsed ultrasound devices.

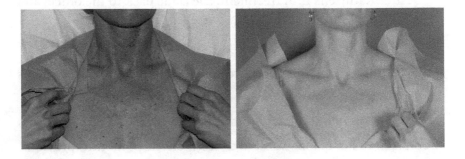

Treatment with intense pulsed light to rejuvenate the skin of the neck and chest.

Energy-based devices really burst onto the photo rejuvenation scene in the late 1980s, when Harvard physicians Rox Anderson and Lawrence Parish proposed a theory of "selective photo thermolysis"; basically, they were trying to create a device that would selectively destroy something in the skin without damaging anything else.[4] So if a dermatologist wanted to get rid of a brown spot or birthmark, he or she could do it without causing injury to surrounding tissue. The first laser invented based specifically on their theory, the pulsed dye laser, was developed for treating port wine stains.

LASER/LIGHT/ENERGY-BASED PROCEDURES
Procedure Totals 2012-2017

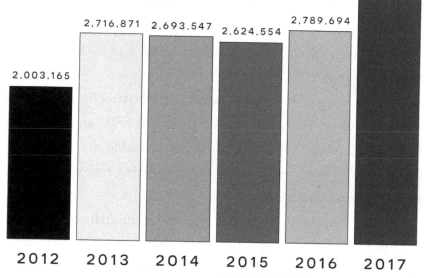

2,003,165	2,716,871	2,693,547	2,624,554	2,789,694	3,274,847
2012	2013	2014	2015	2016	2017

AMERICAN SOCIETY FOR DERMATOLOGIC SURGERY (ASDS)

Survey from American Society for Dermatologic Surgery showing trends in laser and light based devices from 2012 to 2017.

---

4   R. Rox Anderson and John A. Parrish, "Microvasculature Can Be Selectively Damaged Using Dye Lasers: A Basic Theory and Experimental Evidence in Human Skin," *Lasers in Surgery and Medicine* 1, no. 3 (1981): 263-276, https://doi.org/10.1002/lsm.1900010310; RR Anderson and JA Parish, "Selective photothermolysis: precise microsurgery by selective absorption of pulsed radiation," *Science* 220, no. 4596 (April 1983): 524-527, https://doi.org/10.1126/science.6836297.

But most people don't know that port wine stains can be minimized or nearly eliminated. It takes time, but we can lighten them significantly. A few years ago, a patient came to PotozkinMD Skincare Center who had lived her whole life with a port wine stain on her forehead. She was always self-conscience of the mark; she felt it was the first thing people looked at when they saw her. Like most people, she had been unaware that there was a treatment available for the discoloration.

I used a pulsed dye laser device called VBeam Perfecta, which significantly reduced the mark so that it wasn't even visible anymore.

The patient was so happy with the results; she felt a lot more self-confident and didn't think people focused on that spot when they looked at her.

My own experience with pulsed dye lasers dates back to the late 1980s or early 1990s, when I was a resident at NYU and lasers were first starting to take off. I wasn't actually operating the laser—I just pushed the gigantic machine from the operating rooms to the dermatology clinic and back.

When I opened my practice in 1998, I brought in a vascular laser to treat blood vessels, a laser for treating tattoo and pigmented lesions, and a laser to treat hair removal. And I kept them stationary in a room, so no one had to push them around.

As technology evolved, we've added the various categories of devices to the practice, including the IPL. I'm an early adopter of technology, but not a first adopter. I don't usually buy a device when it first comes out; I'd rather let other people experiment on their patients until we know what these things actually do.

Colorations as a result of aging or nature aren't the only visible marks we can minimize or eliminate. We also remove tattoos.

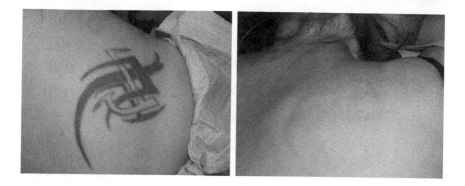

Treatment of a large tattoo with laser. Dramatic improvement with multiple treatments.

In my twenty-five-plus years in dermatology, I've learned at least one valuable life lesson I can pass on to you: Don't get a significant other's name tattooed anywhere on your body. It's okay to have your children's names tattooed, but a girlfriend or boyfriend or even a spouse can end up costing you a very expensive tattoo removal.

It's not uncommon for me to deal with scenarios like this one: A twenty-one-year-old woman who came into my office had her ex-boyfriend's name tattooed across her back. It was a strange, unusual name, nothing common and cool like Jerome. Then they broke up and she wanted to get that branding off. The guy was out of her life, and now she wanted him off her skin, too. His name was in just one color, which made it easier to remove.

We get a lot of tattoos that are just black, and those are the easiest to get rid of. Multiple colors and shades are a little more intensive, but we still get good results with those. Some of the fluorescent ink can be difficult, and in individual cases, there's a chance that we can't completely eliminate the tattoo. We may only be able to lighten it.

We also see people who want tattoos removed so that they can get into the military—you can't get in with a visible tattoo—and people who have large tattoos that they've grown tired of. They want us to lighten that tattoo so they can put something else over it.

Sometimes, though, the reasons for getting rid a tattoo are more significant than a failed relationship or military ambition, such as sex-trafficking survivors who want to erase the name of their former pimp, who branded them as his property by tattooing his name or nickname on her. When the young women escape, they're still stuck with the name on their body.

An organization in Oakland provides those survivors transportation to my office, where I laser those names off at no charge.

When I first volunteered to do this, my expectation was that most of the people we'd be treating would be non-English-speaking women, but that's not the case. Many of these women could be your next-door neighbor.

The technology for tattoo removal was slow to evolve. For years, we used a VersaPulse laser. We used it for so long that its manufacturer stopped servicing it, so I flew in a technician from Arizona to maintain it every so often. But one day, I had three sex-trafficking survivors in for treatment when the VersaPulse went down. Rather than trying to resuscitate it, I went ahead and invested in a picosecond laser, which is what I use now.

Picosecond lasers came onto the market four or five years ago. They emit a high-intensity beam of light energy that is absorbed by the tattoo particles—the ink droplets in the skin—and shatters them into smaller pieces. Different-color lights target different-color ink particles.

Older devices known as nanosecond lasers worked the same, but picosecond lasers do it in far fewer treatments and with less risk. Therefore, while treatment with picosecond lasers is more expensive than with the older devices, it's usually better value because you can remove the tattoo in fewer treatments.

I see a lot of patients for tattoo removal. But the procedure that is in even more demand is skin tightening, which is also one of the most challenging categories, because everybody wants the results of a face-lift without surgery. These devices can't provide that level of rejuvenation. The best expected outcome for wrinkle treatment with these devices is mild to moderate improvement.

When Thermage, the first device for skin tightening, first came out, it was a big deal—the effects of a face-lift in a noninvasive treatment! There was a lot of hype around it because of the desire to tighten skin and give patients the results of a face-lift without a face-lift.

But I noticed something: When I went to conferences, people who were speaking and presenting information about Thermage would show these great, convincing before-and-after photos. But regardless of which physician was giving the talk, they were all showing the same patient's before-and-after pictures.

I think their whole presentation was built around the one person who miraculously responded to the technology, and that person's results were not representative of general outcomes.

So, Thermage wasn't really ready for the mass market at the time it was launched. There were too many bugs that needed to be worked out. The problem was that patients' expectations were set much higher than what we as aesthetic physicians could actually deliver.

As time has gone on, that device has been refined and evolved, and other devices have hit the market. Thermage, a radio frequency device, has improved and is still used for skin tightening. Other such devices for skin tightening have also become available. They all work on the same principle of heating the tissue, causing skin contraction.

There are also devices that use micro-focused ultrasound to heat deep in the tissue, and to heat the layer beneath the skin called SMAS— the layer that plastic and dermatologic surgeons tighten when they do a face-lift. We use one of those devices, called ultherapy.

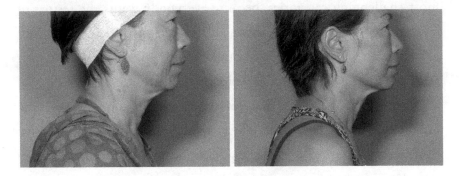

Photos shows skin tightening of the neck before and after treatment with ultherapy (microfocused ultrasound). These results are obtained without surgery.

The drawback with all of these skin-tightening treatments is that we can't guarantee the level of results. No two people respond to treatment the same way, so the results can be somewhat unpredictable. Whereas one person might see significant skin tightening, another might get the same treatment but not the same degree of wrinkle elimination.

I tell my patients about that unpredictability, because I don't want to oversell them on the product or the results. My goal with patient education is that the patient understands the reasons for a course of treatment and the realistic expectations of what that treatment can deliver before he or she makes the decision to go with that option. I strive to match up patient expectation with reality.

With skin tightening, we really want patients to have realistic expectations, but sometimes they don't, and in those cases, they may end up being disappointed with the results.

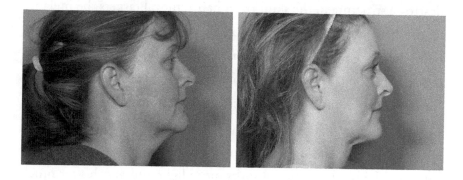

Photos before and after non-invasive skin tightening of the chin and neck.

The next big leap was in laser hair removal. In 1996, one of my former medical school classmates, Dr. Melanie Grossman, published information about using a ruby laser to destroy hair follicles. Since that time, laser hair removal has improved and evolved to become one of the most popular, noninvasive cosmetic procedures.

Most people will need multiple treatments spaced about eight weeks apart. The most common areas women choose to have treated include facial hair, armpits, bikini area, and legs, whereas men usually seek treatment for hairy backs and shoulders.

My goal with patient education is that the patient understands the reasons for a course of treatment and the realistic expectations of what that treatment can deliver before he or she makes the decision to go with that option.

There are many different lasers used for hair removal. They all work on the same principle—using laser light to target and selectively destroy a structure in the skin. Laser hair removal targets the melanin in the hair follicle. For that reason, it works best with coarse dark hair. The more pigment in the hair, the more energy gets absorbed to destroy the follicle. For that reason, laser hair removal doesn't work for light or blonde hair. There isn't enough absorption of the light to heat and destroy the follicle in light hair. It is analogous to an automobile with black interior out in the sun, versus one with white interior. The black interior absorbs more light and gets hotter much faster.

Another advance in lasers that coincided with the popularity of hair removal was the cooling of the epidermis, the outer layer of the skin. Since the epidermis has melanin, we want to heat the melanin in the follicle without overheating the epidermis. If the epidermis is overheated, it can lead to blistering and scarring.

Current laser technology usually has built-in cooling technology where either the laser tip is chilled and comes into direct contact with the skin or the laser has dynamic cooling where a cryogen spray hits and cools the skin just before the laser fires. Because the laser cannot differentiate between the pigment in the follicle and that in the outer layers of the skin, extreme caution must be employed for darker skin types or tan patients. Treating tan and darker skin patients is far riskier than treating non-tanned and fair-skinned patients. The ideal candidate for laser hair removal is someone who is fair skinned with coarse dark hair. This allows us to deliver greater energy with less risk of it being absorbed by the outer layers of the skin and more energy being absorbed by the hair follicle, resulting in a more effective treatment.

Since the advent of the cooling technology, the innovations have been similar to IPL treatment: gradual. At least in the last ten years, there's really nothing radically new in laser hair removal.

But now the market is flooded with energy- and light-based devices for photo rejuvenation of the skin—a variety of devices from many different manufacturers making competing products. Some, like IPL, require little to no downtime.

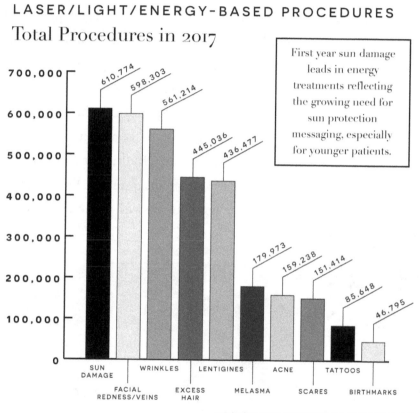

LASER/LIGHT/ENERGY-BASED PROCEDURES
Total Procedures in 2017

> First year sun damage leads in energy treatments reflecting the growing need for sun protection messaging, especially for younger patients.

AMERICAN SOCIETY FOR DERMATOLOGIC SURGERY (ASDS)

This figure demonstrates what laser, light, and energy-based devices were used to treat in 2017. The overwhelming majority of treatments are focused on photo-aging and aging.

Others, like Fraxel Dual and similar devices, are slightly more intensive and require more downtime—usually one or two days. Still others, such as fractionated CO_2 lasers like the Fraxel Repair (which we use in our office), require more downtime, usually seven to ten days. Fraxel was the first innovator to bring "fractionated" resurfacing as a treatment option. Many other device manufacturers have adopted "fractionated" technology, where, as the laser is going across the skin, it is treating multiple tiny "microthermal" treatment zones, which are sort of like pixels on an LCD panel. The energy penetrates into the skin, which the body then repairs by removing the injured tissue. This can result in both improved color and improved texture of the skin. We use Fraxel Lasers to treat skin discolorations, fine lines, and texture irregularities as well as surgical and acne scars. The Fraxel Dual is one of our most popular treatments, as we can get great results with minimal downtime. Multiple treatments are usually required. The fractionated treatments dramatically reduce the risk of loss of pigment that we used to see with some of the older resurfacing devices.

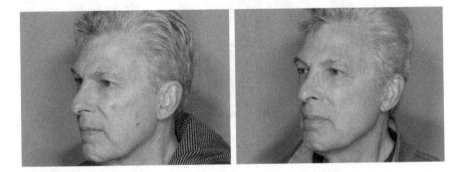

Photos depict a dramatic improvement of the skin before and after treatment with the fractionated CO2 laser.

The more downtime, though, tends to correlate to improved results. So the Fraxel Repair will likely give you better results than the IPL, for example.

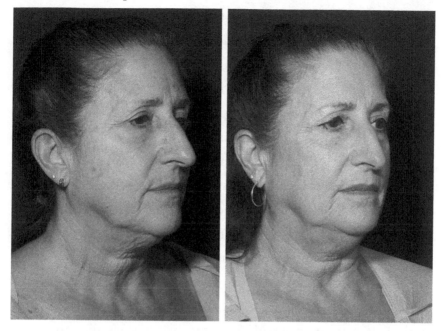

Improvement of skin color and texture following treatment with the Fraxel Dual Laser.

Some of these devices are better than others. And sometimes, as I mentioned, manufacturers rush the devices to the market before we really know what to do with them and how to use them properly. There are some device manufacturers that are known to overstate what their devices can do. They exaggerate the benefits.

So it's really important that you find an expert physician (am I sounding like a broken record yet?) who you trust to vet the devices. Those providers who aren't experts in dermatology or plastic surgery, for example, don't have the experience that breeds a healthy skepticism, or the experience of knowing about the different devices and treatment approaches. They tend to believe it when a sales rep makes those grandiose claims. Then, their clients end up with less-than-promised results.

Unfortunately, I've seen that too often.

I know which vendors are more reputable than others—which ones tend to do the appropriate amount of testing and study—so that's where I start when considering a new device. What I typically do is consider the type of indication we're looking for, whether it's removing brown spots and capillaries or treating wrinkles, and then I look for what I perceive to be the best device on the market based on my extensive research. I will usually speak to colleagues who were involved in the development of the device and have used it firsthand. And then we use it in the office and demo it on staff and volunteers before we bring it on board for patient use.

These devices are usually about $100,000 apiece—so it's uncommon to have every single device in one office. This isn't a big deal, since there are competing devices that do the same things. The provider has to make the call.

And, to be honest, the device isn't as important as the person using it. You can have two different doctors using the same device, and they'll get different results. Most likely, the better result will be with the physician who has more knowledge of how the device works on your specific condition. It doesn't matter if it's the newest and best equipment if the person doing the procedure doesn't really know what they're doing.

The device isn't as important as the person using it.

In fact, it's that way for any course of treatment.

For example, there is a skin condition called melasma, where the pigment-producing cells are working overtime to produce extra pigmentation. There's no static brown spot that you can just zap off with a laser, but rather diffuse brown discoloration. Over the past twenty years, there have consistently been new devices that claim to work for melasma.

But physicians have found that not only do devices not work for melasma the way the manufacturers claimed, but a lot of patients with melasma will actually get worse with laser and light-based devices. The cornerstone of treating patients with melasma is topical medications that suppress the pigment-producing cell, and chemical peeling to turn over the pigmentation.

Ten years ago, I had a patient who had gone to a med spa for treatment of melasma. The nurse there recommended about $6,000 worth of Fraxel laser treatments, so the woman came to us for a second opinion. That was a good decision. I recommended she use a $100 topical cream instead.

She looked at me incredulously, like she was wondering how that simple—and inexpensive—solution could possibly be the remedy to her problem. I told her, "I have the Fraxel laser here in my office. I can give you $6,000 worth of Fraxel treatments if you want, but that's not in your best interest." I have found that people tend to believe me when I recommend things that clearly are not in my financial best interest.

So, she used the topical cream. When she came back eight weeks later, she was about 90 percent better.

Sure, it's in my best financial interest to administer a Fraxel treatment, but it's not in the patient's best interest. And I'm trying to build relationships and recommendations as well as my business. I don't care about one-time payments. I care about lifetime relationships.

And that is what you should care about as well if you're going to invest in any of these energy-based treatments.

CHAPTER TAKEAWAYS:

- Laser and light-based devices really took off in the late 1980s and early 1990s and have exploded since then.

- The key is to choose your expert, not your device, because there are so many devices and manufacturers out there, and it's really hard to figure out what the best treatments are on your own. Go to an experienced professional and trust that they'll do what's in your best interest.

Chapter 4

❧

THE SKINNY ON
BODY SCULPTING

n the early 2000s, two dermatologists at Massachusetts General Hospital, Dr. Dieter Manstein and Dr. Rox Anderson (you may remember him from the previous chapter) had a revolutionary thought. They'd noticed that a young girl who was constantly sucking on a popsicle on one side of her mouth developed a thinner and hollower cheek there compared to her other side.

It was a phenomenon called "popsicle panniculitis," in which infants and young children get swelling and redness in their cheeks after sucking on a popsicle or ice cube. In some cases, popsicle exposure leads to dimples by injuring the fat cells.

Manstein and Anderson believed that meant fat cells are more sensitive to cold temperatures than other types of body cells. So they had the idea to apply that process directly to the fat cells in the human body, and in that way destroy those pockets of fat cells as a way to contour a human body.

That was the origin of cryolipolysis, commonly known as CoolSculpting. Cryolipolysis involves controlled application of cooling within the temperature range of 5 to -11 Celsius to a specific spot on the body to cause cell death of subcutaneous fat tissue, without apparent damage to the overlying skin. The number of fat cells you have in your body is a fixed number; if you can destroy those fat cells, they're gone for good.

Manstein and Anderson tested their procedures on pigs, and the CoolSculpting system was approved for use in the United States by the FDA in September 2010 as a noninvasive alternative to liposuction. The device is extremely sophisticated, with multiple sensors that measure the temperature to make sure there's no damage to the skin.

While the idea was exciting, the initial launch didn't really take off. The manufacturer, Zeltiq, didn't know the best way to use the CoolSculpting system. It came out with a one-size suction cup, but it didn't work well as a one-size-fits-all applicator. It took Zeltiq a while to figure out the best way to use the technology, which isn't unusual for technologies that get out into the marketplace. Often, manufacturers just want to get the device to the market, even if it's not quite ready or they haven't figured out the best way to use it.

Counterintuitively, they figure they'll determine the best way to use it after they get FDA approval.

Seeing those flaws, I didn't initially adopt the CoolSculpting system. I was busy doing a lot of liposuction procedures, which worked really well, and I didn't see the added benefits of CoolSculpting. I also knew there were other technologies coming out, including an ultrasound device being tested in Europe that melted fat that looked more promising to me. When the ultrasound machine got FDA approval, we brought it into the practice and demoed it on three people.

It hurt, they said. It hurt a lot. And, on top of that, I didn't see any appreciable results.

So for me, that was the end of that experiment.

Less than two years later, I was approached by another manufacturer of a different ultrasound technology. They said it could destroy fat, would be pain- and bruising-free, and required no downtime. Someone could be in a bathing suit the next day, they said. At that time, I was researching the best devices for fat-busting on the market and was considering jumping into CoolSculpting, which had evolved significantly by then. But instead, we agreed to become a site to evaluate this new ultrasound device.

We found that most people did not get any noticeable results that they could see in the mirror—and that's the most important consideration with a device like this. It doesn't matter if we can measure with fat calipers and see that there is some improvement. If the patient doesn't see the improvement, it's not worth doing the procedure.

Finally, we made the jump to CoolSculpting. By then, there were multiple applicators, different sizes, different shapes designed for different areas of the body. They were designed to be used in combinations and different patterns, depending on what the person needs.

We brought the system into our practice in 2015. Soon after, we started using it on one of my long-standing patients. We gave her a treatment, and just one month later my nurse called me in to our photography suite to look at her before-and-after photos. My jaw dropped. Her results were similar to the outcomes I was getting with liposuction. I was really surprised, because I wasn't expecting quite that level of change. (Of course, note that this scenario speaks only to the results for that particular patient. For a lot of patients, the results are indeed similar to liposuction without undergoing a surgical procedure, your results might be different.)

If the patient doesn't see the improvement, it's not worth doing the procedure.

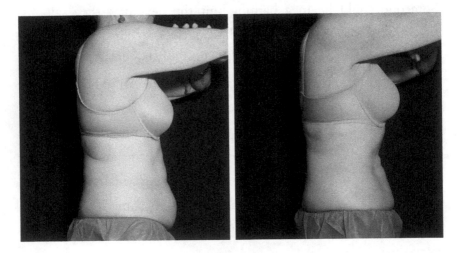

Before and six months after treatment with CoolSculpting to the lower abdomen.

Now, about 99 percent of my patients who are looking to zap troublesome fatty areas request this noninvasive solution.

BODY SCULPTING
Procedure Totals 2012-2017

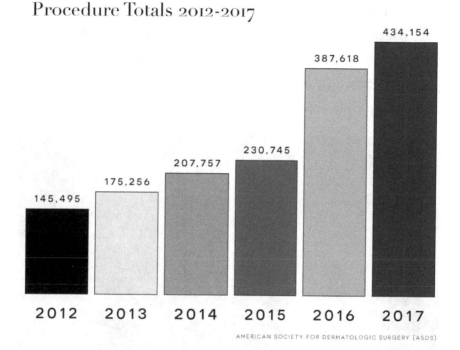

434,154

387,618

230,745

207,757

175,256

145,495

2012   2013   2014   2015   2016   2017

AMERICAN SOCIETY FOR DERMATOLOGIC SURGERY (ASDS)

This figure demonstrates the almost 200 percent increase in body contouring procedures performed from 2012 to 2017. Most of this is because of the effectiveness and popularity of CoolSculpting.

I think the reason it is so popular is, first, that people appreciate a noninvasive option with no side effects and no downtime. Second, CoolSculpting has been available for quite a while now, and there is a lot of consumer knowledge about it. It's certainly the most established body contouring device.

So, when people are thinking of eliminating stubborn fatty spots, they do their research, particularly online, and discover a lot of information about the good and the bad of CoolSculpting.

Then, when they come into my office, we show them photographs of patients we've treated. We're not showing them someone else's patients; we're showing them results that we actually got. It can be pretty compelling. Through the years, we have found that most people are extremely happy with their results, while a very small percentage of people don't respond.

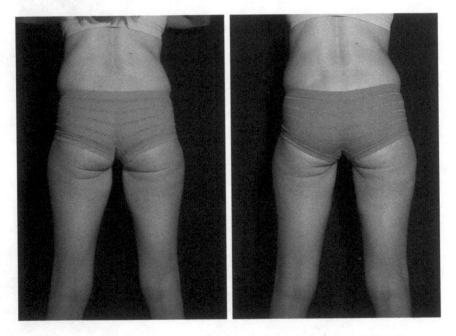

Before and after treatment of the inner thighs with CoolSclupting.

CoolSculpting isn't the only noninvasive body contouring tool. Ultrasound technologies, radio frequency devices, and laser technologies are still out there. And then there is Kybella, which is an injectable that melts the fat. Kybella is used mostly to treat the fat under the chin and neck, called the "submental fullness." I will discuss this in greater detail in Chapter 6. Although the quality of results from the ultrasound technologies are better now than they were when I tested them, a lot of these devices suffer from the same problems I ran into back then—they make claims beyond what the device can do.

So, CoolSculpting is still considered the gold standard, because it works and because of the safety of the process.

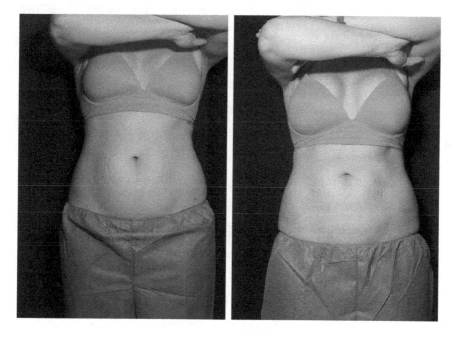

Before and after CoolSculpting of abdomen.

The CoolSculpting procedure is done in thirty-five-minute cycles. We stick the suction cup applicator to the area to be treated, and the patient can watch high-definition TV while the machine does its work. There are no other patients in the room, just one of our nurses popping in and out to check on the person getting the procedure. We can treat up to two areas at a time—that's called "dual sculpting."

The cold, when it hits the skin, can be a bit uncomfortable at first, but after a few minutes the skin gets numb. The suction feels less intense than when you were a kid and you put your hand against the running vacuum cleaner nozzle.

After the cycle, the skin looks like a stick of hard, frozen butter, so we massage it to break the fat cells down. Then we can put the CoolSculpting applicator on another area, if necessary.

When we brought CoolSculpting into the practice, we also invested in another device, called Z Wave, which is used in conjunction with CoolSculpting to get better results. After the CoolSculpting cycle, massaging the area can be really difficult, like trying to massage frozen snow. The Z Wave administers the posttreatment massage with radial pulsed energy. Many believe that using the Z Wave for the posttreatment massage gets better results. We don't charge any extra for this; we just want our patients to get the best results possible.

Since there's no anesthesia, patients can drive themselves to the office and home afterwards. They are not incapacitated in any way. And there's no blood work that they need beforehand.

We can do CoolSculpting on the trunk of the body, arms, chin, inner thighs, outer thighs, bra fat, back fat. There are a lot of options, and they're increasing all the time as manufacturers develop different applicators for different parts of the body.

BODY SCULPTING
Total Procedures in 2017

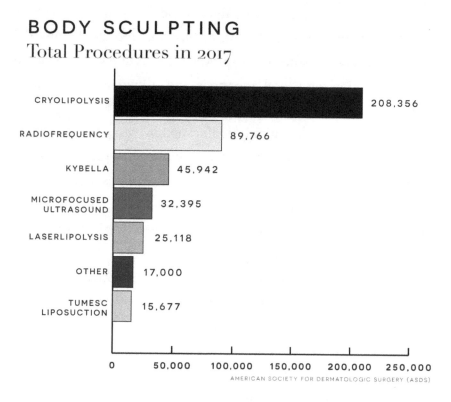

CRYOLIPOLYSIS	208,356
RADIOFREQUENCY	89,766
KYBELLA	45,942
MICROFOCUSED ULTRASOUND	32,395
LASERLIPOLYSIS	25,118
OTHER	17,000
TUMESC LIPOSUCTION	15,677

0   50,000   100,000   150,000   200,000   250,000

AMERICAN SOCIETY FOR DERMATOLOGIC SURGERY (ASDS)

This figure shows the breakdown of body contouring procedures.

Patients can see the results as early as a month out. Typically, the full results will be seen at three to six months—making that early experience I previously mentioned even more impressive.

As I said, nearly all my patients who are seeking body contouring want the noninvasive procedure. But there are still some who ask for liposuction, which I've been doing since the early 1990s.

Dr. Giorgio Fischer introduced the idea of liposuction in 1974, when he used a blunt hollow cannula to extract fat. By the late 1970s, the procedure had become really popular. In 1985, Dr. Jeffrey Klein, a dermatologist, revolutionized the procedure when he invented the "tumescent technique," which involves injecting a large volume of a dilute anesthetic solution that numbs the fat. This constricts the blood vessels, minimizing the risk of bleeding and eliminating the need for general anesthesia. The procedure thus allowed patients to have liposuction with local anesthesia and using smaller cannulas, making it a much safer procedure.

Plastic surgeons historically do liposuction with general anesthesia, which study after study has shown is more dangerous than doing liposuction with strictly local anesthesia. When liposuction is done as a solo procedure—meaning not combining it with multiple procedures with long general anesthesia times—it is very safe. Patients can walk in and walk out of the procedure.

When we do liposuction in my office, we mostly do it completely with local anesthesia in one of our fully accredited operating rooms. A small percentage of people will choose to have some oral sedation as well, but we don't put people to sleep and we don't use intravenous sedation. We do the procedure, which takes anywhere from two to three hours, while people are awake.

The first step is injecting the anesthetic solution. Then we make small, four-millimeter (about a sixth of an inch) incisions in the skin and go underneath the skin with the microcannulas—which are standard, fully tempered, surgical steel tubes—to extract the fat.

After the procedure, there are no stitches. For a lot of patients, the small incisions will heal without scarring. Some people may have a small linear scar, and a very small percentage will form a thick scar.

Then we put a compression garment on the patient. That compression garment is very important—one of the two components needed to get the desired results. (The other, of course, is removing the fat.) The compression garment compresses the areas uniformly and allows the skin to heal and contract.

Most people wear the compression garment for a week, day and night, without taking it off except for showering. Then we have them wear it an additional three weeks during the day when they're up and around.

Most people will see the full results from liposuction in three to six months.

It's important to note, though, that despite the common perception, CoolSculpting and liposuction are not designed as weight-loss techniques. They're not a treatment for obesity. Those procedures are really for people who have localized fatty deposits, areas that they cannot get rid of despite diet and exercise.

It's important to note, though, that despite the common perception, CoolSculpting and liposuction are not designed as weight-loss techniques.

Some patients will come in and say, "Just get rid of all my fat." You can't just get rid of all the fat, though, because fat is important. It brings blood supply and nutrients to the skin.

For patients who come in and need more than a spot here or there treated, I recommend that before undergoing a CoolSculpting or liposuction treatment, they seek nutritional counseling and either start an exercise program or adjust their current one.

What determines whether I perform a CoolSculpting procedure or a liposuction procedure? Some fat can be more tough and fibrous, and that typically does not respond well to CoolSculpting. But usually the choice comes down to simple patient preference. Often, people are willing to pay a little more for the noninvasive treatment.

The cost of CoolSculpting depends on how many cycles a patient needs. If a person has more fatty areas, it will require more cycles. A slim person who has a really small area of fat may just need one treatment; someone who is not close to their ideal body weight and has more fat on their body will require more cycles.

If it's just a couple of small areas, cost can be under $2,000. On average it's about $4,000, because it's not unusual to need more than one treatment.

For nearly all of my patients, the benefits and value of the non-invasive options are simply worth it. Besides less downtime after the procedure, there's also less risk. With liposuction, there's always the potential for infection, bleeding, and scarring, which we don't see with CoolSculpting. When liposuction is overdone, and when it is done with general anesthesia, deaths have been reported. (I haven't seen anything like that, thankfully.) I'm not aware of any such deaths reported with CoolSculpting.

With CoolSculpting, some people will have some discomfort, and maybe tenderness and bruising of the area for a few days. More common is itching. A small percentage will have some diarrhea after the treatment, and a very small percentage (about 0.0051 percent) of people get paradoxical fat hypertrophy, according to the *Journal of American Medical Association*.[5] When that happens, the area that is being treated gets excess fat growth—the exact opposite of what we're trying to do. Researchers are not sure why that happens, and the only way to get rid of that excess growth is to liposuction the area.

We've done hundreds of CoolSculpting procedures, and so far, none of my patients have suffered that side effect. Knock on wood.

---

5   Jalian HR et al. "Paradoxical adipose hyperplasia after cryolipolysis." JAMA Dermatol 150, no. 3 (2014) :317–319, https://doi.org/10.1001/jamadermatol.2013.8071.

As I mentioned, CoolSculpting permanently destroys the fat cells. But the threat of destroying too many fat cells isn't really a concern. The smart technology is designed to measure the temperature of the skin to prevent that kind of injury—unless someone is being treated with an applicator that is oversized for the area being treated.

That means not just anybody should be operating the device. If your treatment isn't done correctly, it won't be effective, or if the wrong CoolSculpting applicator is put in the wrong area, you can have denting of the skin that can be a permanent deformity.

So, as always, I advise you to choose carefully who will perform your procedure. Look for someone who has done a lot of the CoolSculpting or liposuction procedures and has staff who have been properly trained. In California, you have to be a licensed physician, physician assistant, or registered nurse to be legally able to operate the CoolSculpting device. A receptionist isn't able to do that—legally, anyway. Look for a place that has more than one machine, so you can be treated in less time, and that uses the Z Wave, which in my view is a must have for the quality of the procedure.

You want to make sure that your treatment plan is devised by someone who has knowledge and training and knows what they're doing, and you definitely want to see photographs of people who have been treated at that facility. Don't settle for images with a different doctor's name at the bottom. Make sure the name at the bottom is the name of the physician you're meeting with so that you can be sure those are results he or she actually obtained.

Only accept the best for your money and your body.

CHAPTER TAKEAWAYS:

- CoolSculpting is safe and effective. For some people, results can be similar to liposuction surgery.

- But as with any procedure, you want to make sure you're having it done in a facility where they know what they're doing and have experience and expertise doing it.

- You'll have better odds of getting a favorable result if you're having your procedure done in a dermatology or plastic surgery office rather than at a dental clinic or a facility where a non-aesthetically trained doctor is the supervising physician.

Chapter 5

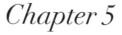

FOR WOMEN ONLY

By guest author Dr. Monica Brar

I t may seem odd that Leslie came to PotozkinMD Skincare Center for help with vaginal dryness and discomfort when she had intercourse. She was in her late forties, had given vaginal birth twice, and had an autoimmune disease that contributed to her issues. As a result, she didn't look forward to having sex anymore, which was definitely affecting her relationship with her husband.

She'd also noticed some vaginal looseness ("laxity" is the term we use), and her tampons weren't staying in as well as they used to. In certain yoga positions, she had the sensation of air passing out through her vagina, and when she coughed or sneezed, some urine occasionally leaked out.

In another case, Diane, in her mid-fifties, complained of some urine leakage with coughing and sneezing, which was becoming annoying and on occasion required a pad. She didn't want to do "anything drastic" to treat it, as she had a friend who had undergone surgery for incontinence with suboptimal results. She also didn't want to have to deal with wearing pads. She had some mild vaginal dryness, which she could live with, but the urine leakage not so much.

The vaginal dryness was even more acute for fifty-nine-year-old Elise: "Another word in my head for intercourse is pain, because it's just so dry, and we use lubrication, and it doesn't help," she told me. Oral estrogen would have helped, but she was reluctant to take that because it increases the risk of breast cancer, which ran in her family.

It might not seem like a dermatologist's office is the place to go for these problems. But at PotozkinMD Skincare Center, we specialize in rejuvenation, and what they—and many others—were looking for was a noninvasive form of vaginal rejuvenation. Our office also has the advantage of having me on staff, as I was a board-certified obstetrician gynecologist before I transitioned to treating leg veins. So it was natural for me to perform and supervise these vaginal rejuvenation treatments.

Vaginal rejuvenation is a catchall phrase to describe a wide range of different therapies and procedures designed to improve the health and function of the vaginal tissue and turn back the clock a bit. At one end of the spectrum are those treatments that are the most benign, which include over-the-counter lubricants to help with vaginal dryness in women who have gone through menopause and who are dealing with postmenopausal vaginal changes such as thinning of the vaginal tissue, decreased lubrication, itching, burning, and frequent bladder infections.

Then there's hormone replacement therapy, which can range from vaginal estrogen that's delivered via a vaginal tablet, to vaginal rings that patients can insert and leave in, to vaginal creams, patches, oral pills, and other delivery systems, all offering different degrees of systemic absorption into the bloodstream.

Vaginal rejuvenation is a catchall phrase to describe a wide range of different therapies and procedures designed to improve the health and function of the vaginal tissue and turn back the clock a bit.

For patients who suffer from loss of urine, another option is Kegel exercises, which strengthen the pelvic floor muscles that support the bladder and other pelvic organs. Until recently, the next step up in treatment was surgery to repair the structural issues, such as lifting the bladder if it is protruding into the vagina and causing urinary incontinence. But surgery has its own set of risks, requires anesthesia, and has a recovery period.

Now, though, there are energy-based devices that can stimulate vaginal rejuvenation without surgery. They fill the gap between hormone replacement therapy and surgery nicely. (Many women affected by these issues have not gone through menopause yet, so their options for treatment are even more limited.)

These energy-based devices deliver either laser or radio frequency energy (depending on the device) to stimulate new collagen formation in the vaginal mucosa lining and increase blood flow to the area. The end result should be that the tissue is a little tighter and a little stretchier, has increased tone, and, with the increased blood flow and collagen, should be much better lubricated.

Ablative lasers such as Mona Lisa Touch and FemLift stimulate the collagen by vaporizing the outer layers of the skin; non-ablative lasers, such as IntimaLase and Petit Lady, and radio frequency energy devices, such as Geneveve, Thermi, ThermiVa, and V-Revive, heat up the targeted tissue without actually destroying it. The significant difference between the lasers and the radio frequency energy devices is that the latter penetrate deeper into the mucosa. Therefore, lasers require more treatments than procedures done with radio frequency devices.

Dermatologists have had radio frequency and laser available to treat tissue and skin, and somewhere along the way, someone noticed that those devices had a gynecologic application to improve collagen formation and help with vaginal tightening and tone. In 2014, the Mona Lisa Touch became one of the first such energy-based devices to enter the market for this procedure.

But I was skeptical. I do the leg vein procedures at PotozkinMD Skincare Center, but as a former practicing OB-GYN, I was thinking, "Are people really going to pay $3,000 [the cost for the procedure] just so they'll be more lubricated?" I didn't think enough people would be interested to justify the cost of the equipment, and since I hadn't practiced in the field for a few years, I didn't have any patients to talk with about it. It certainly wasn't something the patients I performed vein treatments on had complained about.

Then I started researching the procedure and I found quite a lot of information online. These devices have flooded the market. The Kardashians and one of the Real Housewives, according to the internet, have had these treatments done. Vaginal rejuvenation treatment is often talked about on the morning talk shows and has been mentioned in popular women's magazines. As the procedure has entered mainstream media and our collective awareness, interest has grown and women are talking about it. This is especially true in the demographic that I see for my vein practice, which is composed mostly of women who have had children.

After mentioning it to some of my long-standing leg vein patients, I realized that the desire for this kind of treatment was more pervasive than I'd thought. Soon, I realized that this new procedure—noninvasive and nonsurgical, with no medica-

Vaginal rejuvenation treatment is often talked about on the morning talk shows and has been mentioned in popular women's magazines.

tion required and very minimal side effects, if any—could make a huge impact in patients' private lives.

As an OB-GYN, I'd seen many patients who would have benefited from this technology. I certainly saw patients who were either around menopause or had gone through menopause and were experiencing vaginal atrophy (the drying out of the vaginal tissue), but who didn't want to take hormones because they were fearful of potential side effects. Back then, though, we were limited in what we could offer: There were over-the-counter lubricants that can help to some extent but do not improve the elasticity of the vaginal wall. There was also the option of a vaginal estrogen product that works locally with minimal systemic absorption. Some women were hesitant to use vaginal estrogen creams because they were messy, and some felt the vaginal estrogens did not help enough to alleviate their symptoms. So there was really no good answer for those patients.

This, though, could be the perfect answer to that problem. It's ideal for treating a wide range of issues:

- It can help improve vaginal tone and tightness in women who have had vaginal births in which the vagina tissue gets stretched out, leading to decreased sensation with intercourse, decreased enjoyment with intercourse, or the sensation of tampons slipping out.

- It can help women suffering with vaginal dryness during intercourse by helping to build new collagen in the vaginal walls, which improves blood flow and increases lubrication.

- It can improve the elasticity of the tissue, making intercourse much more comfortable and enjoyable for menopausal women suffering with dryness and discomfort.

- Once estrogen level decreases in menopause, the vaginal tissue tends to get thin and dry, and this can help restore some of that without the patient having to take hormone replacement therapy.

- It can help women suffering with mild to moderate stress urinary incontinence via new collagen production and without the need for a major surgical procedure.

So, in 2017, after researching all the devices on the market, we invested in the Geneveve radio frequency device, which either I or our female physician assistants perform. We selected the Geneveve because it has a higher radio frequency than the other devices currently on the market, raising tissue temperatures more quickly. It also uses a higher wattage of power for greater therapeutic effectiveness in a single treatment. The Geneveve offers cryogen cooling to protect the vaginal mucosa, which the others don't offer. The Geneveve can hold higher tissue temperatures (50-55 degrees Celsius) for longer before quenching the treatment area with the cooling, whereas the Thermi system, for example, shuts off the power when only 42 degrees Celsius is reached, and there is no active cooling. The Geneveve also penetrates much deeper into the foundational layers of the vaginal tissue than other devices on the market.

Besides the basic science of how the Geneveve device works, it is the only technology with positive clinical results for sexual function and vaginal laxity from clinical trials. Viveve (the company that created the device) is the only company in the United States with an ongoing FDA Investigational Device Exemption (IDE) trial for improvement in sexual function. It is important to note that both the FDA and other global regulatory agencies only grant approval to conduct human clinical trials if there is extensive safety testing. Viveve has been able to demonstrate that, with the Geneveve device, there is no injury to vaginal or surrounding tissue. Canada just approved Viveve to conduct a clinical trial in Canada into its use in the treatment of stress urinary incontinence. And as of today, there are no known device-related, serious adverse effects reported in any ongoing or completed studies with the Geveveve device.

In July of 2018, the FDA took action against several companies who market devices for vaginal rejuvenation due to safety concerns, however, Viveve was *not* one of the companies included. This, no doubt, has everything to do with Viveve's commitment to patient safety, research to back up their results, and their proven clinical benefits.

So when Leslie, Diane, and Elise came into our office, we had the tool to help them.

When a patient calls with interest in the Geneveve procedure, the receptionist schedules her a complimentary phone or face-to-face consultation. The patient completes a questionnaire to determine whether she has issues that the Geneveve will be able to address and that we will review together. If she's in the office, I'll do a pelvic exam to assess whether she's a good candidate. If it's a phone consultation and the patient seems to be a solid candidate, we schedule the procedure and do a quick pelvic exam before the procedure to confirm.

A number of patients have told me during the consultation that when they mentioned to their husbands or partners that they were considering this procedure to help with intimacy issues, their significant other was all for it. Currently, it is not a procedure that is covered by insurance, but it is a procedure that both partners can benefit from.

The procedure takes about sixty minutes. The patient lies on the exam table with her feet in the stirrups and a grounding pad on her leg (since we're using electrical energy). The treatment tip that actually gets placed inside the vaginal canal is about the diameter of a thumb. It's relatively small and easily tolerated, and on that little thumb, where the thumbprint would be, is a one centimeter by two centimeter surface through which the radio frequency energy is transmitted.

With some lubricant, the treatment tip is gently inserted into the vaginal opening. The vaginal wall just inside the hymenal ring is circumferentially treated all around with the exception of the 12:00 position right under the urethra. A total of 110 pulses of radio frequency energy are delivered in thirty minutes. Then, that treatment tip is removed and a longer tip is inserted in the same gentle way, and another round of 110 pulses of energy is delivered several centimeters deeper into the vaginal canal (thus making the total treatment time sixty minutes and 220 pulses).

Each pulse is delivered over seven seconds, and in that time, the Geneveve delivers the radio frequency energy into the vaginal mucosa. It also simultaneously cools the vaginal mucosa as mentioned above. With each pulse, a patient may notice a tolerable warm sensation, and that should be the worst of it. (I have had patients work on their laptops and take phone calls during treatment.)

After treatment, the patient can resume all her normal activities. The only thing we ask of her is to avoid intercourse or tampons for forty-eight hours. It is not uncommon for patients to have a little bit of discharge for a couple of days. Other than that, it is business as usual.

Because it takes about thirty days before the new collagen will start to form, we tell patients, "Don't expect to see much in the first month." At about thirty days, they should start to notice a little bit of a difference, but it takes ninety days for the full effect of new collagen formation and improved blood flow, and thus improvement in stress incontinence, lubrication, tightness, and other results.

I call all patients about thirty days out just to see if they've noticed anything, and then I have them come back in ninety days so that we can talk face-to-face about the results they've noticed.

Not every woman is a candidate for the procedure, though. Those with an implantable electric device such as a pacemaker or an automatic implantable cardioverter/defibrillator are absolutely NOT candidates. We also don't want patients who are taking anti-inflammatory medications on a daily basis, because those drugs can affect collagen production and diminish the results. We don't want to do the procedure on someone who is breast-feeding or has been breast-feeding in the last six months, because that can also affect the results, since breast-feeding reduces estrogen levels.

Of course, we don't want to do the procedure on someone who is pregnant, or someone who is planning to get pregnant in the upcoming six months. And we want to wait six months after chemotherapy or radiation therapy so that we can give the patient the best chance of getting a good outcome from the vaginal rejuvenation.

Not every woman is a candidate for the procedure, though.

Leslie was a perfect candidate for the procedure, as was Diane. Elise was a good candidate, although not perfect. At the time of this writing, Elise is still early in her three-month window for seeing results, but Leslie was one of the first women we treated. Six months out, she no longer needed to use a lubricant. Her husband could tell things were tighter down there, and she said her tampons stay in better. While she still experiences a little loss of urine, that has definitely improved, too. We were able to address almost all of her issues with the treatment, and it impacted her relationship, as sex is now much more pleasurable. Diane, in turn, is thrilled with her results, telling us that three months after treatment she had no loss of urine despite coughing from a nasty case of the flu.

We know from studies by Millheiser[6] and Sekiguchi,[7] respectively, that a year after treatment, approximately 90 percent of women

---

6   LS Millheiser et al., "Radiofrequency treatment of vaginal laxity after vaginal delivery: Nonsurgical vaginal tightening," *J Sex Med* 7, no. 9 (September 2010): 3088–95, https://doi.org/10.111/j.1743-6109.2010.01910.x.

7   Y Sekiguchi et al., "Laxity of the vaginal introitus after childbirth: Nonsurgical outpatient procedure for vaginal tissue restoration and improved sexual satisfaction using low-energy radiofrequency thermal therapy," *J Womens Health (Larchmt)* 22, no. 9 (September 2013): 775–81, https://doi.org/10.1089/jwh.2012.4123.

have achieved significant and sustainable results in sexual satisfaction and the integrity of the vaginal tissue. We look forward to getting the results of the ongoing studies to determine how long lasting the results will be.

There's a general perception that a lot of what dermatologists do is about vanity, and to some degree, the Geneveve procedure can be about cosmetics as well. It can treat the outside of the vaginal opening—the outer lips or labia minora and majora. We have treated a handful of patients, women in their late forties and early fifties, who have had vaginal births and felt like the labia had gotten stretched out and misshapen and no longer looked the same. In this era of Brazilian waxes and laser hair removal, women are more aware of and sensitive about the external appearance of their vaginal opening. The Geneveve, by helping to stimulate collagen formation and tighten tissue, can be a nonsurgical way to help shrink down the labia and improve the aesthetic appearance to a more youthful one.

But for most, Geneveve is about improving functional issues—helping them experience less discomfort, more pleasure, and a decrease in the loss of urine.

While the procedure isn't cheap, it is a one-time treatment to treat current problems. We don't have any long-term data to know exactly how long the results will last, but patients may elect to have it done again eventually.

From a medical standpoint, it's a safe procedure with no reported risks in the studies. One of my concerns was if a patient is not already complaining of vaginal looseness, or, conversely, if they feel they are on the tight side, are we going to overtighten? There were no complaints about that in the studies, but the studies were done on women who'd had vaginal births, so further research is needed to evaluate a broader range of patients. I recently spoke with a physician who has extensive experience with the device and who has done some of the research, and I asked him that question. In his experience with similar patients, he reported seeing no overtightening, but rather improved elasticity and therefore improved function and sexual satisfaction.

As with any procedure, it's important that the patient select an experienced provider with knowledge in the field. Conversely, it is important for the provider to accurately assess the patient before performing the treatment to be sure she's a good candidate. For example, I've had a few women come in who were interested in the procedure to treat severe stress incontinence. But their cases were so extreme they needed to see a urologist for surgery; I did not feel Geneveve was going to make a big enough difference for those women and referred them out.

From a medical standpoint, it's a safe procedure with no reported risks in the studies.

One of our regular patients expressed interest in the procedure. She was in her late forties, had no children, was not sexually active, and had stress urinary incontinence. She wore a pad, but she felt the leakage wasn't that bad, and she had not yet seen a urologist for it. She was interested in a procedure that could help reduce or alleviate her leaking problem with minimum risk and downtime. After getting her history, I proceeded with an examination to determine if she could benefit from the Geneveve treatment.

Over time, the tissue that holds the bladder up and away from the vagina can weaken. When I do the pelvic exam, I can see how much the bladder protrudes into the vaginal canal when someone coughs or sneezes or bears down. When I asked this patient to cough, the urine came out not as a leak, but as an arching stream that soaked my pant leg. Her bladder protrusion was significant.

The Geneveve can help a little with that, but not enough to fix this woman's problem. I'm confident in saying that had I done the procedure on her, any improvement would have been negligible. The Geneveve isn't going to take the place of having surgery to lift the bladder, and that was clearly what she needed.

"I'm so sorry to tell you this, but you need to see a urologist," I told her. She was appreciative of me telling her that, because she would have gladly spent the money if there was a chance that it would make a noticeable difference.

Without that exam, without looking specifically for that problem, and without the background to know to look for that problem, a provider may have just performed the vaginal rejuvenation procedure anyway. This patient would have been out that money, and still would have needed surgery (and the additional costs of surgery) immediately.

Med spas and other pop-up clinics, though, sometimes concern themselves less with whether the patient is a good candidate than with whether their check will clear. Sometimes they're not doing what's best for the customer—they're doing what's best for their bottom line. I would like to think that there are ethical and informed providers in those establishments, but the stories I hear from patients do not always support that assumption.

So, even though there's little medical risk from the procedure, you will be best served by going to a facility that has a licensed doctor or appropriately trained provider on the premises. These procedures are only as good as the person performing them. You want that person to be able to tell you if it's worth your time and money for this treatment or if there's a better option. Seeing someone for a vaginal rejuvenation procedure who is not well versed in at least the basics of gynecology and who doesn't understand the pelvis will decrease your odds of getting a treatment that you will be happy with. These are elective procedures not covered by insurance, so you want to invest your money wisely. And typically, elective procedures do not come with a money back guarantee if you do not get the results you were expecting.

At PotozkinMD Skincare Center, we make sure that you're a good candidate, or we won't take your money to do the procedure.

Med spas and other pop-up clinics, though, sometimes concern themselves less with whether the patient is a good candidate than with whether their check will clear.

As with anything, it is difficult to guarantee a particular result, but we do our very best to deliver and therefore screen patients carefully.

There is steadily growing public interest in vaginal rejuvenation, and there are an abundance of energy-based devices for performing it, but there is not a lot of research yet. Many studies are ongoing with the Geneveve device to help us as physicians modify and improve these treatments to further improve effectiveness. I look forward to the results to help me better counsel and treat my patients.

But for now, when done by the right person and for the right reasons, this treatment offers significant benefits. When you're considering getting the procedure, make sure you're a good candidate based on what you read in this chapter. It might have worked for someone else, but before you invest your time and your money, do your research to determine if it will work for you as well.

There's so much information available online, and having a little bit of a background will help when you initially meet with the provider. Also, it will help you have realistic expectations of your outcome. Spend time with the provider weighing the risks and benefits, discussing possible outcomes.

If you educate yourself, and request information and education from your provider, you're much more likely to be happy with the results of your procedure. Remember, while 90 percent of patients in the studies mentioned earlier in the chapter had improvement, 10 percent of the women weren't all that happy with their outcome. When you're spending your money, you want to do everything you can to increase your odds of ending up in that 90 percent group.

> *There's so much information available online, and having a little bit of a background will help when you initially meet with the provider.*

CHAPTER TAKEAWAYS:

- Just like skin, the vaginal tissue is made up of collagen. As women age, collagen weakens, and many women begin to experience a decrease in vaginal tightness, lubrication, and sexual arousal. Intercourse may be painful, and stress incontinence is common.

- In recent years, the market has been flooded with nonsurgical vaginal rejuvenation devices to restore that collagen and diminish or eliminate the bothersome symptoms with minimal risk.

- We have elected to offer the Geneveve radio frequency device for vaginal rejuvenation over all the other technologies currently on the market because it's very well tolerated, it consists of only one treatment (unlike all the others, which require multiple treatments), it offers simultaneous cooling so a higher temperature can be achieved and therefore deeper tissue penetration, it has no significant side effects when used appropriately, and it has solid science to back up the results.

Chapter 6

⌒

NOT FOR WOMEN ONLY

Women, hand the book over to your husband, boyfriend, brother, father, or any other significant male in your life. I want to talk to him for a few minutes. Rejoin me for Chapter 7.

Hey, man, I know it's a bit embarrassing to admit that you need to get cosmetic work done to look your best, but more men than you realize do just that—and there's really nothing to be embarrassed about. Gender-specific data from the American Society for

Aesthetic Plastic Surgery showed an increase from 772,000 nonsurgical cosmetic procedures for men in 2005 to over 900,000 in 2014.[8]

Nationally, five to ten percent of cosmetic treatments are administered on men.[9] It's a growing trend. (But the female aesthetic market has been growing a lot more rapidly than the male aesthetic market.)

In my practice, about five percent of cosmetic patients are men. They come in for Botox to eliminate a permanent angry scowl, to smooth out lines, and to fill in the hollows on their face to help them look younger to compete in a tough job market. My office is near Silicon Valley, and the technology industry is becoming a younger person's game, so these guys in their forties and fifties feel like they need to look younger.

Or they come in seeking help for stubborn love handles, a weak chin, and an excess of back and shoulder hair.

Half the time, they're being dragged in kicking and screaming by their wife or girlfriend. There are a couple of reasons for this male reluctance, I think. One is societal pressures. Historically, from the time women are little girls, they've been judged on how they look, and men are judged on how much money they make and how successful they are. I'm not saying that these are my beliefs; it's just the way things have been from a historical perspective. There's a lot of pressure ingrained in women to look their "prettiest," but that's not a measurement of men.

Also, women are much more likely to talk about these procedures with their girlfriends. If you look at advertising for these

---

8   CS Frucht and AE Ortiz, "Nonsurgical cosmetic procedures for men: trends and technique considerations," *J Clin Aesthet Dermatol* 9, no. 12 (December 2016): 33–43, https://www.ncbi.nlm.nih.gov/pmc/articles/PMC5300725.

9   "2017 Plastic Surgery Statistics Report," American Society of Plastic Surgeons, https://www.plasticsurgery.org/documents/News/Statistics/2017/plastic-surgery-statistics-full-report-2017.pdf.

aesthetic procedures, it's almost all geared toward women. It's only been in the past year or two that we've seen Botox, Xeomin, and Dysport starting to gear some advertising campaigns toward men. It is just now that we are hearing about things like "Brotox."

Women talk about this stuff with their girlfriends when they're getting their nails done, when they're in the hair salon, or sharing a bottle of wine. When men get a procedure, they don't tell anyone; they don't want anyone to know.

NEUROMODULATORS

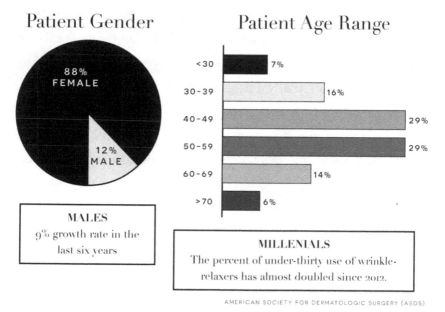

This figure demonstrates the increase in neuromodulator treatments such as Botox, Xeomin, and Dysport in men.

There's still a social stigma when men get these procedures, but it's becoming more acceptable as men realize the career benefits of looking fresher and younger.

No matter how they end up coming in, the men who get procedures in my office are nearly always happy they did get the work done—and they nearly always come back for the regular follow-up procedures. They become loyal patients.

For example, Oscar's girlfriend sent him to my office for Botox because he had that permanent scowl I mentioned earlier. She thought he was angry and mad even when he wasn't. But it wasn't just his girlfriend who felt that way. He worked in real estate sales, and others had mentioned that he always looked angry. That certainly didn't help in a competitive real estate market.

We injected his "glabella frown lines," the creases that made him look angry, with Botox. A week later—that's how long it takes for Botox to take full effect—the lines were gone, and people started reacting to him differently. His girlfriend didn't feel like he was angry at her. He noticed his sales numbers went up by about 34 percent, which is something I have seen among salespeople when Botox flattens out their frown lines and people perceive them as being friendlier.

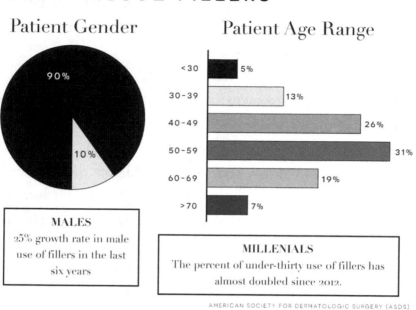

SOFT-TISSUE FILLERS

Patient Gender

Patient Age Range

This figure shows the increase in filler use among men.

Oscar was really happy with his treatment, and now he comes back every four months for maintenance.

Injecting men is different than injecting women, because men's faces are shaped differently than women's faces, so there are a lot of considerations the person doing the injections has to consider. With Botox, which relaxes muscles, men usually have bigger, stronger muscles in their face, so they may need a slightly higher dose than women. If you look at a man's face, their brows tend to be lower and more horizontal than women's. You definitely don't want to feminize a man's face.

Treating men is different in another way, too. Men don't want people to know they're getting enhancements, so they can't have the bruising or other telltale marks from a procedure.

I'd say that we see some bruising with fillers around 20 percent of the time. With Botox, it's unusual to see bruising. But any time you're sticking a needle into the skin where there are little blood vessels, it's possible to have bruising.

So sometimes guys will wait until they're going on vacation to schedule their appointment so that they will be away from coworkers and others for a scheduled period of time. (But if the procedure is poorly done, it's very possible there will be bruising that will still be noticeable more than a week later.) In addition, there are things we can do to minimize bruising—avoiding aspirin, for instance, and some people will take a supplement called Arnica that can minimize the risk of bruising.

If someone does have bruising, we will treat them with a pulsed dye laser, which can make bruises go away faster. And then there are different makeups and cover-ups. But whereas women have no problem putting those on, usually men feel very awkward and uncomfortable.

They're already going to a cosmetic shop, and now we're putting makeup on them? That may be a little over-the-top.

Although aesthetic procedures for men haven't been socially acceptable for the most part, they have been mainstream for more than thirty years. It started with Rogaine, which was approved by the FDA in 1988. Before then, men would get hair transplants that looked horrible, with clumps of hair sprouting from the head like a poorly made doll. It was often so obvious that the eye got drawn to the plugs. If it looks like you've obviously had something done, you're better off not doing anything—particularly if you're a guy.

There have been significant advances in this area, and instead of putting plugs in, doctors are doing single hair grafts. That can look completely natural, but it's extremely time intensive.

In 1997, the FDA-approved Propecia, an oral medication designed to restore hair loss. That was a big deal, because it was more effective than Rogaine and easier since it was just one pill a day.

Those hair restoration procedures really opened the door for other procedures for men. (Check out Chapters 2, 3, and 4 for more on those other procedures.) We're now smoothing wrinkles, filling in hollows, and even removing hair.

The revolution that started with men trying to regain lost hair has now evolved into men trying to get rid of hair. Laser hair removal works really well for permanently shaving away that heavy, dark, course hair on the back and shoulders.

There's also a big male market for CoolSculpting. A lot of guys we see are into fitness. They want to look and feel their best. So they'll exercise daily and slim down—but a lot of times there are certain stubborn areas of fat on their body that they just can't get rid of despite diet and exercise. Usually, it's the love handles and lower abdomen.

Doctors can get rid of those fatty deposits with lipo-suction, but CoolSculpting has

The revolution that started with men trying to regain lost hair has now evolved into men trying to get rid of hair.

really taken off as the preferred treatment for many. We get great results with it. It's nonsurgical. It's noninvasive. Guys can come in, have a treatment while they're hooked up to the machine watching ESPN on a big flat-panel television, and be back at work the next day—with those trouble spots no longer a problem.

Here's the good news: CoolSculpting actually destroys those fat cells, so they won't come back. (Chapter 4 has more on body sculpting.)

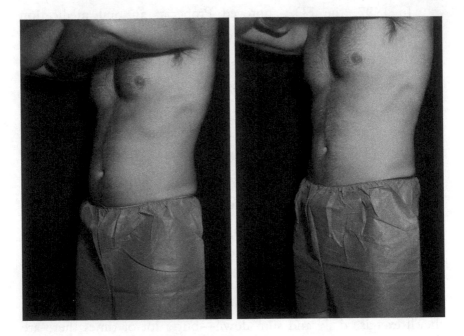

*Before and after treatment of the love handles with
CoolSculpting. This area is extremely popular for men.*

That's how it worked for Eric. He was fifty-five and in really good shape, and he worked out regularly, but he hated taking off his shirt because of his love handles. They really bothered him, but genetically, he could not shake those pouches. He was a great candidate for CoolSculpting, so we performed the thirty-five-minute procedure.

A month later, Eric came back to the office for his follow-up. When we looked at his pictures, wow—I wouldn't say we were surprised, but we were really pleased about how great a result he had. Then, when we saw him at his three-month visit, he was telling us how he loves going in the swimming pool. He likes taking his shirt off now.

That response is pretty standard.

I would say probably 20 percent of the CoolSculpting treatments we administer are on men—so if that's something you're considering, you're certainly not alone. More often than not, again, in my practice at least, it's their wife or girlfriend sending those guys in.

Another thing that often drives men crazy is having this fat under their chin, the double chin, or what we call "submental fullness." Historically, the only real treatment option for that was liposuction. However, in the last couple of years, there have been big advances in that arena. In 2015, the FDA approved an injectable drug called Kybella. The active ingredient, deoxycholic acid, permanently melts fat. When patients seek treatment with Kybella, they usually require three to six treatments, depending on how much fat they have. I like to inject a local anesthetic before the Kybella because it really stings if you don't numb the area first. The biggest downside with Kybella is that there can be quite a bit of swelling that typically lasts about a week. When we melt the fat, some people worry that the skin is just going to sag where the fat had been—but that's not the case. Rather, the skin naturally contracts, so you're not left with turkey neck. This treatment is also very popular with women.

In addition to Kybella, CoolSculpting is an option for some people. The CoolMini CoolSculpting applicator is designed for treating the submental fat. We just stick it on the underside of your chin for half an hour and let it freeze away the fat.

While the percentage of women I see for most procedures is significantly higher than the percentage of men, there's one exception to that: laser tattoo removal. With men, it's usually for one of three reasons: to remove an ex-girlfriend's or ex-partner's name; to erase visible tattoos so that they can join the military (the military has strict rules about not having visible tattoos); and to erase or lighten

While the percentage of women I see for most procedures is significantly higher than the percentage of men, there's one exception to that: laser tattoo removal.

old tattoo designs that they've gotten tired of and want to put something new on top of.

If you want to know the truth, one thing that I've learned in twenty years of practice is that, counterintuitively, women are much braver than men. Women are oftentimes fearless compared to men, and can tolerate a lot more. When we're injecting a woman, often she won't bat an eyelash, whereas when we do the same procedure on a guy, he's likely to wince and express his discomfort or pain.

(I'm the same way. I stick needles in people's faces all day long, whether I'm injecting local anesthesia or filler or Botox. But I went to the dentist to have a cavity filled recently and I was stressed out. Is this going to hurt? I felt like a little kid again.)

So, when we're treating men, we take a slightly different approach. I usually take baby steps. I like to prioritize things based on what's bothering the guy and stay focused on the main area that brought him in. Then, going forward, I branch out and expand our educational process.

And with men, I focus on the procedures and equipment that will minimize downtime.

No matter what procedure a guy is having, the key is that it provides natural-looking results, not overdone and not poorly done. Because men are often looking for stealth, under-the-radar procedures that will make them look better without anyone noticing or knowing what they've had done, it's critical for you men out there to go to someone who's really experienced and knows what they're doing—someone who will take the time to educate you and take things one step at a time, instead of trying to accomplish everything all at once.

That will increase the likelihood of a great outcome.

CHAPTER TAKEAWAYS:

- More men are undergoing aesthetic procedures because it's becoming more socially acceptable.

- Men typically get cosmetic procedures for different reasons than women. They usually do it to be more competitive and to stay relevant and current in their career.

- Men can experience significant improvements to appearance and self-esteem with properly chosen procedures performed by experienced providers.

- Men tend to prefer proceeding slowly through potential treatment options versus doing every potential treatment at once.

- With men, less is more.

Chapter 7

⸺

SO, HOW SHOULD YOU CHOOSE A PRACTITIONER?

W hen I was a basketball-playing teenager, I really wanted a pair of Adidas SuperStar basketball shoes. But they cost more than $30, which was beyond my family's budget. Then one day, my dad, a school vice principal, came home excited: he'd bought a pair of sneakers that looked just like the SuperStar sneakers that I was yearning for, but he'd bought them for a mere $10.

These less-expensive shoes would soon gain a reputation as being a great bargain—as long as you didn't mind having bleeding feet. I wore them for three days and then had to put on more comfortable sneakers.

That's when I learned that deals that are too good to be true are just that: they're never really that good, and very often they end up costing more in the long run. With most things in life, we get what we pay for.

It's the same with rejuvenation procedures. Too often, people respond to an offer for cheap procedures that seem too good to be true. And they almost always are.

For example: Jennifer went to a med spa for a discounted Botox treatment. On his website, the doctor boasted about how he trained other dermatologists in cosmetic procedures at the annual American Academy of Dermatology (AAD) meetings, so he seemed a great option for her procedure. Then, after her Botox, he pressured her to also get sclerotherapy to get rid of blood vessels around the eyes.

Too often, people respond to an offer for cheap procedures that seem too good to be true.

Sclerotherapy is a procedure in which a sclerosant solution is injected into a blood vessel to destroy it. It's commonly performed to treat leg veins; however, injecting it in the face has the potential to leave permanent scarring and has resulted in blindness when injected around the eyes, a possible side effect that was not disclosed to Jennifer.

It's a procedure that I don't do on the face, and the recommendation for that procedure was wrong on many different levels.

By those standards, I guess Jennifer got lucky. The needle just opened a large gash on her face. But the on-site doctor couldn't treat the wound, and his advice for treating it actually made it worse.

Fortunately, with time and a handful of noninvasive pulsed dye laser treatments, Jennifer healed with barely a mark on her skin. But treatment required about three weeks of wound care to get the skin to heal back over, and then eight weeks of laser treatments to erase the scar.

She later discovered that the doctor who performed the procedure was neither a dermatologist nor a plastic surgeon, but rather a family practitioner. He lied about his credentials on his website and had never actually taught other dermatologists cosmetic procedures.

When I contacted the AAD, I was told they'd never heard of the doctor, and that he'd never spoken at any AAD event. The organization sent him a cease-and-desist letter to stop him from making that claim. But for Jennifer and his other patients, the damage had been done.

Then, there's another doctor in Southern California who does these treatments, and on her website, she claims she's double board-certified by the American Board of Dermatology and the American Board of Pathology, and subtly suggests that she's a dermatologist. But if you look deeper into her website, you learn that she did one year of internal medicine and did her residency in anatomic pathology. Then she did a fellowship in dermatopathology, looking at biopsies.

In truth, then, she has no clinical training in dermatology whatsoever.

But she's practicing dermatology now.

That's audacity.

As I've said throughout this book, these procedures are pretty safe and offer great value if they're done by the right people. But how do you know who is legitimate and who's not?

In this chapter, I hope to educate you about the various settings in which one can best receive noninvasive cosmetic procedures so that you can make an informed decision. I'll tell you what to look for, what questions to ask, and what to avoid. This will by no means be a guarantee that you will have a great outcome with minimal risk, but it will dramatically put the odds in your favor.

It starts with understanding that most, if not all, of the minimally invasive cosmetic procedures that are so popular today were developed and perfected by physicians who received training in what are known as the "core four" aesthetic specialties. These physicians typically completed residencies and are board-certified in dermatology, plastic surgery, otolaryngology (ENT), or oculoplastic surgery. As part of the residency in these specialties, the physicians learn the foundation of knowledge necessary to safely and effectively perform noninvasive cosmetic procedures.

As we've discussed, though, the rising popularity of noninvasive cosmetic procedures has led to a corresponding rise in medical professionals entering this arena. That has led to the rise of the med spa.

Your best option is still to get the procedure from a doctor trained in one of the "core four" specialties. No matter where you live, there's very likely to be highly trained, board-certified dermatologists, plastic surgeons, ENTs, and oculoplastic surgeons nearby who can evaluate your aesthetic concerns, educate you about your options, and safely and effectively treat you.

So why go off the beaten path?

Nearly every time I see a patient who has had a botched procedure, that patient had the procedure performed in a less favorable setting, such as a poorly supervised med spa. In truth, it causes me to scratch my head. I can't understand why those patients didn't seek out a highly trained specialist.

Of course, the "core four" physicians are not immune to complications, as complications will occur even in the most skilled and trained hands. However, it is important that any complication be recognized early and treated appropriately, and they know how to do that, too.

I get that these med spas might be attractive because of convenience and possibly lower prices. However, you may be

Nearly every time I see a patient who has had a botched procedure, that patient had the procedure performed in a less favorable setting, such as a poorly supervised med spa.

putting yourself in danger, and in the long run, you may end up spending more when a costly mistake is made and you need to pay for corrective measures.

Many of my colleagues might be surprised to learn that I don't necessarily think it's wrong for a family practitioner to enter this arena. I do believe there are many highly intelligent and very capable non-core physicians who have gotten the training and education to do this competently.

But there are too many med spas where there is no physician supervision other than a "supervising physician" listed on a piece of paper who is never really there. Many med spas have a supervising physician in name only, with a doctor renting out his or her license and never actually being on-site, and oftentimes having no training in the procedures they are supposed to be supervising. There have been cases of rectal surgeons, anesthesiologists, radiologists, and even psychiatrists supposedly supervising these facilities. They're getting paid a monthly retainer because the med spa needs a physician of record. There's no supervising going on.

For example, I just got an email for a promotion at a hair salon where there's a nurse doing injections and the supervising physician is a radiologist. A radiologist, even if he or she is actually on the premises, doesn't have the specialty training to perform these procedures.

If someone is a family practice doctor claiming to be a dermatologist, that shows they're a dishonest person. Would you choose a dishonest person to be your doctor? The blatant distortion of one's credentials to the point of fraudulently representing oneself is unethical. It's important that they honestly and ethically present their education and background, or they don't deserve your business.

If you choose to go to a med spa for minimally invasive procedures such as injectables or laser procedures, you will be best served at a med spa that is either part of a physician's office or one that has direct on-site supervision with a physician who has appropriate training to supervise the treatments and manage any complications. These treatments are not without potential risk, and you need someone there who can identify a possible complication and treat it. No matter how trained, a nurse is probably not going to have that knowledge.

With some of these treatments, you legally need to be evaluated by a physician. The injectables are all prescription drugs or medical devices, and if you're not being evaluated by a physician, that clinic is engaging in unlicensed practice of medicine. (At least, that's the case in the state of California.)

If you insist on going to one of these med spas, don't just jump in. Get your information from the spa, do your independent research, and then go back to have your procedure.

When you visit the clinic to inquire about a procedure, ask:

- Who is the supervising physician, and when is this physician on-site?

- Who will be performing the procedure and what is their education and training? Regulations on who is allowed to perform different procedures varies by state, but there are frequently limitations. In California, for example, injectables and laser and light-based treatments can only be performed by a licensed medical professional such as an MD, PA, or RN.

- What are the physician's credentials? Is the physician board-certified? What are they board-certified in? Board certification means that after residency, they passed a lengthy and rigorous test to demonstrate competency. That training will give you a greater likelihood of having a better outcome.

In California, if a physician claims to be "board-certified," he or she must legally state what they're board-certified in. Otherwise, a psychiatrist could claim to be "board-certified" and limit their practice to dermatology, and an unsuspecting patient would assume they are board-certified in dermatology.

So, it's a giant red flag if you see a physician claiming to be board-certified but not stating what their board certification is in. Another red flag is a physician listing the institutions where they did their residency training but not stating what their residency was in.

Ask these questions at the clinic, and then go do independent research on Google. You can get pretty far on your own there. You can double check their certification by looking it up on the American Board of Medical Specialties website (www.abms.org). Look up the doctor on your state's medical board website; do they have any complaints against them?

And please, please, don't ever get an aesthetic rejuvenation procedure in a salon or someone's living room. Those settings are wrong for so many reasons. Remember that these are medical procedures and should be performed in a clean medical environment. A hair salon or someone's living room is not the place you want to receive your treatment.

So, it's a giant red flag if you see a physician claiming to be board-certified but not stating what their board certification is in.

In an online professional group that I'm a member of, one of my colleagues posted an article about two RNs who come to the patient's home and administer Botox, filler, and vampire facials (a combination of microneedling and platelet rich plasma). The supervising medical director is a cardiologist and husband of one of the nurses. They call themselves a "concierge service."

"How is this legal?" my colleague asked.

Good question.

When procedures are performed outside of a physician's office, all bets for safety and results are off. You're more likely to be injured or burned. If actual surgery is being performed in one of the fringe, nonlicensed places, you're actually taking your life in your hands. You don't truly know the credentials of the person performing the injections or know exactly what they're injecting. There are many sad cases of people dying after getting injections outside of a medical setting.

For example, in 2014 a woman in Georgia was convicted of depraved-heart murder (legally defined as an action that demonstrates a "callous disregard for human life" and results in death) after a woman she injected with silicone butt injections died from a blood clot in her lung a few days later.[10] In September 2017, a New York woman was arrested on manslaughter charges after a mother of two died twelve days after she received silicone butt injections. A medical examiner said she died from complications of systemic embolization of silicone injections (silicone getting into the blood vessels).[11]

While death is an extreme case, there are plenty of other complications that can happen in those settings. I've seen it many times in people who have come into my practice. Many of those people have told me they had a gut feeling that something was off but didn't want to hurt someone's feelings.

Remember, *it's your face and body*, so don't worry about someone else's feelings, especially when that person is trying to exploit you. There are times when you need to take care of yourself more than the other person. Don't worry about the doctor's feelings; he or she will live. Follow your gut.

While we're on the subject of the doctor performing the procedure, don't discount the doctor's innate aesthetic awareness. There is an art to this, and an injector who has a grasp on what makes a face look more natural and fresher is a big advantage for you.

---

10   Mary Bowerman, "Woman convicted in fatal buttocks-injection procedure dies in prison," USA Today, January 16, 2018, https://www.usatoday.com/story/news/nation-now/2018/01/16/woman-convicted-fatal-buttocks-injection-procedure-dies-prison/1035294001.

11   "Woman Arrested In Silicone Buttocks Injection Death Faces Arraignment," CBS New York, September 29, 2017, https://newyork.cbslocal.com/2017/09/29/silicone-buttocks-injection-death.

For example, for years I took sculpting classes at a university in San Francisco to train my aesthetic eye. Now when I'm working with injectable fillers, I know that I want to sculpt the face in such a way that there are highlights and shadows, just like when I'm building an art piece and I'm adding clay to build up a certain area. It's the same thing, only now, instead of clay, I'm adding hyaluronic acid into the skin to build up areas where there's a volume deficit.

It definitely helps to blend the artistic, creative eye with the scientific body of knowledge.

How can you know if the doctor you're talking with has that eye? Your own eyes are the best source for determining that. When you're in the office, pay attention to the people working there and what they look like. If you walk in and all the women working in the office have distorted, overdone features, that might not be a good thing.

There is an art to this, and an injector who has a grasp on what makes a face look more natural and fresher is a big advantage for you.

If they all look natural and fresh, you can have confidence that the doctor has a good aesthetic eye.

The last two decades have seen an explosion of amazing, minimally invasive cosmetic procedures. Laser and light-based devices have progressed significantly. Injectables such as neuromodulators and fillers have revolutionized how we can turn back the clock on aging. With all of the tools in the aesthetic physician's toolbox, you should be able to get a great and natural look. However, it is extremely important that you do your homework on where you receive treatment and who is performing the treatments.

Remember, there are credentialed professionals who have extensive medical training in these procedures, and one (or more) of them is very likely within a short drive of where you live. These procedures are the core of what they do, not some service they added onto their main business as a way to make more money.

By going to them for your procedure, you increase the likelihood of a great outcome with minimal risk.

On the other hand, when you go the cheaper route, very often the cheaper results are apparent. And then you'll end up spending more money in the long run to correct the problems from the poorly performed procedure. And, of course, because those doctors or nurses are just doing this for the added money, they'll often try to up-sell you for procedures you don't even need, so then you end up paying more than you intended—with decreased results.

It's your face and your body. Treat it like a temple, and invest in the best value. After all, you don't want to end up with a gash on your face or blood in your knockoff shoes.

CHAPTER TAKEAWAYS:

- Have your cosmetic procedure done in a physician's office, or at least at a med spa that's part of a physicians' office and has on-site physician supervision.

- You want the physician to be board-certified in one of the "four core" aesthetic medical specialties: dermatology, plastic surgery, ENT (ear, nose, and throat), and oculoplastic surgery.

- You get what you pay for. If it looks too good to be true, it probably is.

- Don't jump right in. Do a little bit of research on your own and make sure that what you're being told is legitimate. Google is your friend, and with a little bit of work you can find out pretty much anything you need to know.

- If you have a gut feeling that something is wrong in that facility, heed that instinct.

Conclusion

⁓

When a person is considering getting a cosmetic rejuvenation procedure done, they often worry about whether they'll look strange or different. And they're concerned about the risks involved.

But if you go to the right physician for the procedure, you minimize those risks and maximize the chances that you'll get great results. Looking natural is the key, and everyone has a different philosophy on what that means and how to achieve it. My philosophy is that we want people to look like the best natural version of themselves and not look overdone. Most people don't want to be overdone. Some do, but I'm not the right guy for them.

Picking the "right guy" (or woman) is essential to getting great results. You want the right synergy between yourself and the person doing the treatments. If you pick the right provider and then go into the consultation with a little bit of knowledge about your options, and if you know enough to be able to determine if the provider is trustworthy, and if you can get that synergy with him or her, you increase your chances of a great outcome.

Hopefully, the information in this book will help you understand those options, what to look for in the office and online, and what questions to ask if you're seeking to look your best without undergoing surgery.

My single most important piece of advice is to choose the expert, not the device. There is no "one size fits all." There are many options out there. There are many different injectables that all have their own properties, and there are literally hundreds of devices. I love Google, but it is not possible for someone without expert knowledge to figure out what is best for them. So you'll be best served seeking the care of a true expert who can evaluate your needs and educate you about the various options.

All of these treatments, whether they're injectables or treatments with devices, tend to be safe and effective; however, there's no such thing as a risk-free treatment. That does not exist.

Risks and complications can happen in the best of hands, the most highly skilled hands. But when procedures are performed by someone who hasn't gone through the training for board certification, or who has been inadequately trained, complications are more likely to occur. And, as we've seen several times in this book, when they do occur, those nurses or undertrained doctors aren't likely to have the education to know how to take care of the problems. Then you're forced to come to someone like me to deal with the disaster, and suddenly that savings you thought you were getting has become expensive—in money and in time off work.

If it seems too good to be true, it most likely is. You get what you pay for. Pick the cliché. They're trite, but they're clichés for a reason.

Now, I'm not saying that the only people who can correctly perform these procedures are dermatologists or plastic surgeons or ENTs, because I do think there are excellent nurse injectors out there. There are excellent physicians who are not dermatologists or plastic surgeons who can do these procedures well. But it's really important to vet these people to make sure they're not making false claims and that they're set up to immediately deal with any complications.

If you want to come see me, I welcome you. I'm a board-certified dermatologist, which means that after medical school, I did residency training specializing in dermatology. When I completed my residency, I did a fellowship at UCSF in dermatologic surgery, where we were exposed to a lot of different cosmetic procedures, different lasers, and so forth. I have been a teacher at UCSF, where I train the next generation of dermatologists. I have been a trainer for some of the major laser companies and the major neuromodulator/filler companies. I've also won many awards for my work.

My overall practice philosophy is to treat everyone as if they were a member of my own family and create relationships for life. That's my goal.

I leave you with a final thought—perhaps an odd thought coming from a dermatologist, but an honest thought: For most people, some of the little things that bother them appearance-wise are only apparent to them. Most other people don't even notice minor imperfections. The procedures I wrote about in this book are great, but don't get overly consumed with them and overly caught up on perfecting your looks.

Accept yourself for who you are.

But if you want to look like a fresher version of you, do your research.

Good luck with your procedure(s). I hope I see you soon.

Our Services

We proudly offer all medical dermatology procedures in addition to the following cosmetic procedures.

For more, visit **Potozkin.com.**

COSMETIC DERMATOLOGY

LASER SURGERY

BODY CONTOURING

INJECTABLES

MOHS SURGERY

MEDICAL DERMATOLOGY

About the Author

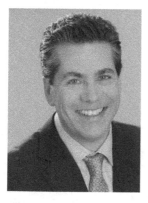

JEROME R. POTOZKIN, MD, is the founder, practitioner, and CEO of PotozkinMD Skincare Center. This center has over ten thousand patient visits per year and is a fully accredited outpatient setting accredited by the Institute of Medical Quality (IMQ). Patients travel across states for treatment—even as far away as Hawaii.

Dr. Potozkin is a board-certified dermatologist and fellowship-trained mohs surgeon. He has been named to San Francisco's "SuperDocs" on multiple occasions. He is the recipient of the prestigious Sulzberger Prize at The NYU Skin & Cancer Unit. He has been quoted in the New York Times and has been feature on national television on shows such as ABC's 20/20 and NBC's Today Show as an expert in cosmetic dermatology. He has been published in multiple medical journals. He is one of two dermatologists to serve two terms as the president of CalDerm and currently sits on their board of directors. He has served as the section chair of dermatology of the John Muir Medical Center. He teaches future dermatologists at UCSF. In 2016, his facility was chosen as the first SkinCeuticals Advanced Clinical Spa in California. He served on the board of directors of the Association for the Accreditation of Ambulatory Health Care (AAAHC) from 2009–2015. In 2005, he founded "Vanity for Charity" in response to Hurricane Katrina and has since raised tens of thousands of dollars for local and national charities. He was awarded the 2017 "Business Person of the Year" by the Danville Chamber of Commerce for his contributions to the community.